hathayoga

rey devereux

photographs by clare park

Thorsons

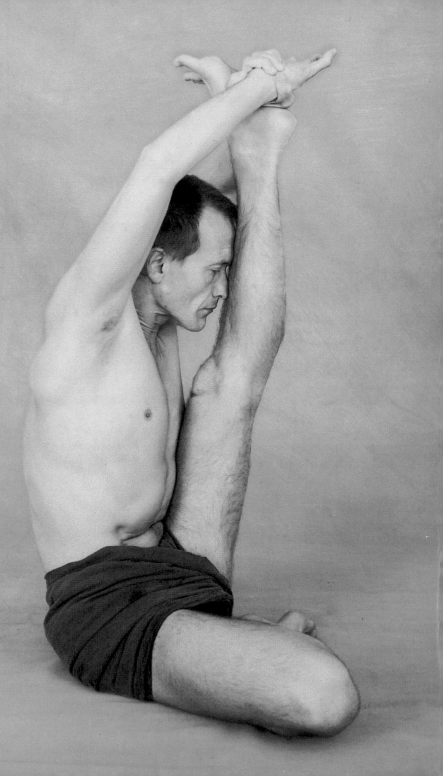

Thorsons
An imprint of HarperCollinsPublishers
77–85 Fulham Palace Road,
Hammersmith, London W6 8JB

The Thorsons website address is: www.thorsons.com

10 9 8 7 6 5 4 3 2 1

Editor: Jillian Stewart
Design: Jacqui Caulton
Production: Melanie Vandevelde
Indexer: Susan Bosanko

Godfrey's website address is: www.windfireyoga.com

All photography © Clare Park

A catalogue record for this book is
available from the British Library

ISBN 0 00 710310 7

Printed and bound in Singapore for Imago

contents

Acknowledgements   v

Welcome   vi

Introduction   1

    The context of hatha yoga   3
    The simplicity of hatha yoga   6
    How to use this book   11
    Practical considerations   14

Lesson one: Relaxation   17
Lesson two: The foundation   31
Lesson three: The core   49
Lesson four: The bandhas   59
Lesson five: Engaging the arms and hands   77
Lesson six: Engaging the legs and feet   87
Lesson seven: Moving with the breath   101
Lesson eight: Using the legs   113
Lesson nine: Adjusting the pelvis sideways   129
Lesson ten: Adjusting the pelvis forwards   143
Lesson eleven: Straightening the legs   157
Lesson twelve: Releasing the spine   171
Lesson thirteen: Softening the back   189
Lesson fourteen: Strengthening the spine   201
Lesson fifteen: The art of stillness   213

Extra shorter practices   222
Index   226

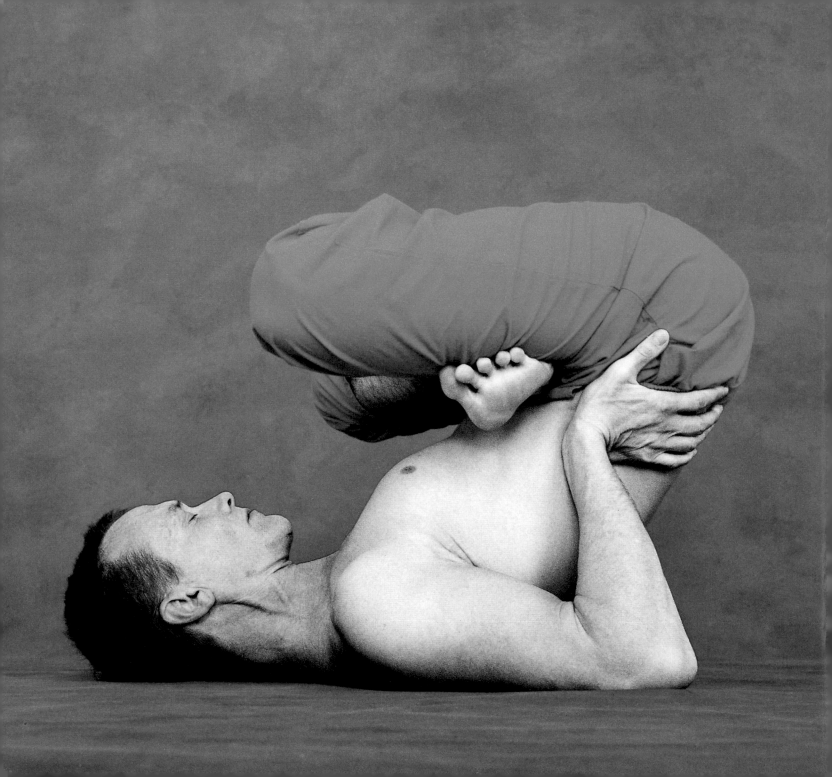

This book is dedicated to

B.K.S. IYENGAR
'the lion of Pune'

for providing me with such sure and solid shoulders upon which to stand

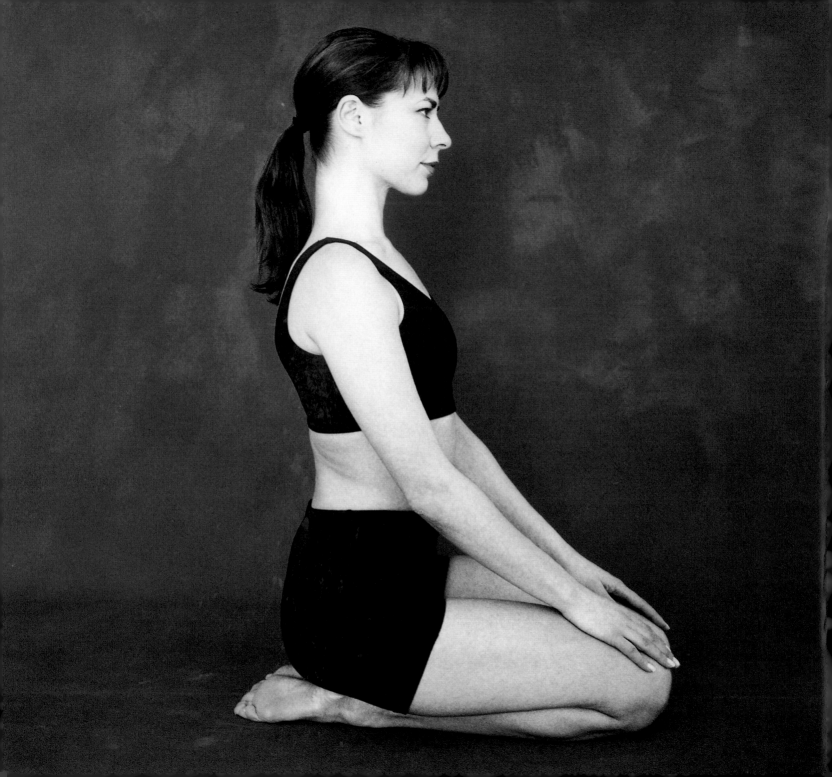

This book is for everyone who wishes to experience the deep and lasting benefits of yoga practice. While the lessons it contains are designed to take an absolute beginner to accomplished self-practice, they will equally benefit more seasoned students.

This book constitutes a single whole. Please read the first part before attempting the lessons. Begin with the first lesson and proceed slowly to the next in sequence only when you have become stable and comfortable in all of the postures of that lesson.

No matter how experienced you are, approach this book with an open mind and it will reward you.

Every moment of your life
every event that you participate in or witness
every word you hear or read
can enrich you
if you meet it fully, openly
and with love

For more on the technicalities of the yoga method please consult *Dynamic Yoga*, also by Godfrey Devereux. For a variety of shorter practices please refer to the author's *15 Minute Yoga*.

Caution

This book does not constitute a therapeutic or remedial manual. If you are ill or injured please consult a medical professional with a practical understanding of hatha yoga, and a yoga teacher trained in the therapeutic application of the method.

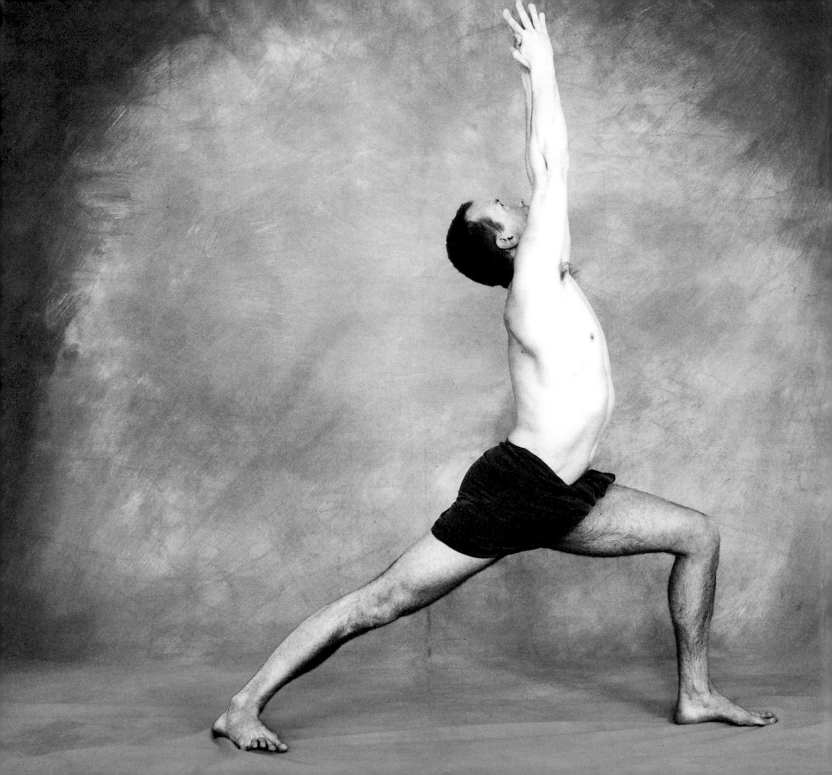

Yoga is not a physical fitness system. It is not a religion, a cult, a New Age fad. It requires no strange beliefs: no blind faith. There is no need for penance, confession, humiliation or self-denial. It is not a way of life with a predetermined set of values and conventions. You do not need to burn incense or wear prayer beads. You do not need to give up onions, meat, tobacco, alcohol, sex or money. Hatha yoga is a spiritual practice. It is a means of clarifying that which is, and expressing it directly, fully and harmoniously. It is, then, both a science and an art. There is rigour, objectivity and revelation in its method. There is harmony, beauty and inspiration in its expression.

In practical terms yoga involves the release of the human potential. This means the full power of your body and the full power of your mind become available. The deeper you go into the practice, the more this potential will fulfil itself. From the very beginning, however, you will notice greater relaxation and calmness; increased freedom of movement; improved balance; enhanced concentration and alertness; increased self-confidence, determination, contentment. These can be felt even after one session. It is these practical and immediate benefits that will inspire further practice.

The way that we make the shapes of hatha yoga demands that we let go of the habitually limiting ways that we use our minds and bodies. They insist that we break out of the old, set patterns that restrict us. They free us from our dependence on the known, the familiar. They allow us to feel safe and comfortable in the unfamiliar, the unknown. In doing so they make available that which lies beneath the patterns of restriction that limit and define us. They bring us in touch with the deeper potential that lies dormant within. Releasing this potential is not a process of construction. It is not even one of dismantling. It is one of enquiry and acceptance that brings about a spontaneous shift in our way of being. We no longer identify ourselves with the superficial, transient, partial and circumstantial movements, sensations, feelings, thoughts, ideas and beliefs that give us a sense of unique separateness. Instead we allow them all to have their temporary place, to fulfil their momentary brief, without losing sight of the greater whole of which they are but a small and passing part.

This is the meaning of yoga, union. It brings about union of the different, splintered aspects of ourselves. Within this union each of the different parts is empowered, validated and uplifted by its relationships with the others. This process occurs on many levels. Union of movement and breathing; union of muscle and muscle; union of bone and bone; union of the anatomical and physiological bodies; union of the peripheral and central nervous systems; union of mind and body; union of thought and action; union of desire and intent.

This is the purpose and function of yoga. To give us what we are, as a whole. It is not about becoming more flexible, stronger, fitter, or any other external benefit. These things are simply incidental, rewarding side effects. However, if we focus too much on achieving them we can miss the whole point. If our mind becomes narrow in its external ambition it will become neither stable nor comfortable enough to bring about union. For ambition creates a tension in the mind that disturbs it. Union requires a spacious, accommodating mind that can tolerate all of the different aspects of ourselves – aspects that can often appear to be in conflict when not set within the harmonizing context of the whole.

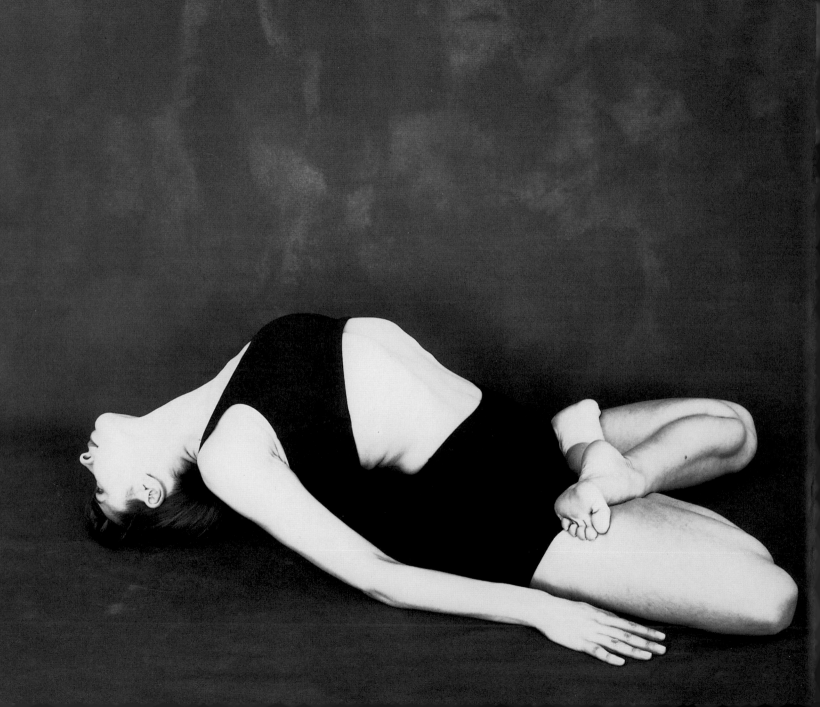

The practices of hatha yoga must be approached in a very definite way if they are to bear their intended fruit. This has been defined by Patanjali, regarded as the root guru of classical yoga. He outlines five attitudes and five orientations (known as yama and niyama), the context in which they occur (asana), and their effect when applied there (pranayama).

'sensitivity, honesty, openness, focus, and generosity are yama.' yoga sutras II. 30
'commitment, contentment, passion, self-reflection and devotion are niyama.' yoga sutras II. 32

'they generate love, fulfilment, abundance, vitality, freedom from identification, detachment, independence, integrity, joy, presence, freedom and self-knowledge, peace of mind, purification, awareness of the infinite and the highest realization.' yoga sutras II. 35–45

'joyful steadiness in the body free from tension and manifesting the infinite beyond duality is asana.' yoga sutras II. 49–53

'within asana, pranayama is the release of inhalation, exhalation and transition till they become unhindered and subtle through exhaustive interpenetration until the duality of the breath is transcended, uncovering the inner light and readying the mind for meditation.' yoga sutras II. 49–53

The practice of hatha yoga must be undertaken without violence (ahimsa). This means to be sensitive to the limitations of body and mind while challenging them. Hatha yoga is not a question of bludgeoning our way through our limitations. It is a matter of challenging their presence until they naturally dissolve in the light of our awareness. Sensitivity is absolutely essential to a physically safe practice. The hatha yoga postures require use of muscles, tendons, ligaments and joints that are totally unfamiliar. To rush into them with only the goal in sight is potentially dangerous. We must be willing to find our limitations before we can recognize them.

The practice of hatha yoga must be undertaken with honesty (satya). This means utilizing all of the resources that we have while practising, and not pretending to those we have not. If we can straighten a leg, we do so. If we can ground our feet then we do. If we cannot, then we do not try to force it. Honesty is absolutely essential to a psychologically safe practice. Without it we can push ourselves deeper and deeper into the anxious tyranny of divisive ambition, and become more and more deeply cut off from what we actually are. We must be willing to recognize our limitations before we can release them.

The practice of hatha yoga must be undertaken with openness (asteya). We must not be full of predetermined ideas about what we will or want to find. These will only serve to deflect us from what is actually present. Of course we will have some to begin with. But as we practise we can learn to let go of them. Wanting more (of whatever) from our practice is an expression of poverty-consciousness. Trying to get more when it is not naturally there is a form of attempted theft. We must be willing to accept our limitations before we can release them.

The practice of hatha yoga must be undertaken with focus (bhramacharya). We must not disperse or waste energy. We waste so much energy when we try to force our body into positions for which it is not ready, or try to impose rhythms and qualities on our breath for which it is not prepared. To push for more drains us, slowly but surely. Equally wasteful is to allow the mind to wander away from what we are doing. Daydreaming is the antithesis of yoga. We must be willing to focus on our limitations in order to release them.

The practice of hatha yoga must be undertaken with generosity (aparigraha). We must not resent what we find when we practice. We have spent years using and abusing our bodies and minds in a narrow range of habitual ways. It takes time to change this. We must be willing to honour our limitations if we are to release them.

These five attitudes are not really separate. To be gentle we must be honest, to be honest we must be open, to be open we must be generous, to be generous we must be focussed. They interrelate with one another end-lessly, creating a mindset without which the practices of hatha yoga will be limited. They must be applied within an orientation that also has five interrelated aspects.

The practice of hatha yoga must be undertaken with total commitment (sauca). Yoga is a challenging process. We must do what we do without hesitation, hedging or holding back. We must dedicate all our energy, all our attention, all our effort to our practice. Total commitment to what we are doing in every aspect brings purity to our practice. Without this purity it will yield sour fruit.

The practice of hatha yoga must be undertaken with a content willingness (samtosa). Our practice must be without resentment, anxiety or doubt. We must be inspired by love for what we are doing: not by desire for the results it might produce.

The practice of hatha yoga must be undertaken with burning enthusiasm (tapas). If our practice is not enflamed by a passion for life, for discovery, for being, it will be impossible to maintain our commitment and our contentment when faced with the many difficulties opening to ourselves inevitably entails.

The practice of hatha yoga must be undertaken as a process of self-enquiry (svadhyaya). Self-enquiry is the heart of yoga. Its techniques are nothing more or less than potent mirrors for profound self-reflection. Any other motivation will lead to limited and possibly distorting and troublesome consequences.

The practice of hatha yoga must be undertaken in a spirit of devotion and gratitude (pranidhana). Although devotion cannot be fabricated and is generated by authentic practice, it is our fundamental safeguard. The techniques of yoga are potent generators and amplifiers of energy. Whatever we bring to our practice will be enhanced and expressed. To be sure that it is not our petty ambitions, fears, desires and egoism that are amplified a sprit of genuine devotion to the sanctity of all that exists is a prerequisite.

Yama (attitude) and niyama (orientation) are the indispensable context within which asana (yoga posture) and pranayama (yoga breathing) mature via pratyahara (meditative internalization) into the heart of yoga: dharana (meditative concentration), dhyana (meditative contemplation) and samadhi (meditative absorption). These are the eight limbs (ashtanga) of classical yoga praxis.

Hatha yoga is a very powerful but simple process. It is simply a question of using the body to free the breath. The breath is the dynamic link between body and mind. Hatha yoga then is about using the body to transform the mind through the agency of the breath. We begin to free the breath by freeing the body. As the body opens, relaxes and stabilizes within harmonious muscular relationships, the breath is released and the mind opens and stabilizes. The arena of yoga then is the postures.

THE YOGA POSTURE

The definition given to yoga posture (asana) by Patanjali is succinct but clear.

'yoga posture is comfortable (sukha) stability (sthira) in the body free from tension manifesting the infinite beyond duality.' yoga sutras II. 46,47,48

Only when the body is free from tension is it capable of being genuinely comfortable and stable. And only then is it capable of manifesting the infinite beyond duality. This quality is the context and trigger for meditation. It occurs when our attention is no longer caught by sensations that distinguish right from left, front from back, inside from outside. Then the body no longer makes itself felt as a finite limitation. Then our attention is brought quite naturally to the breath. This is the root of meditation.

'within asana, inhalation, exhalation and transition become unhindered and subtle through exhaustive interpenetration until the duality of the breath is transcended uncovering the inner light and readying the mind for meditation through pranayama.' yoga sutras II. 49,50.51,52,53

THE METHOD OF YOGA POSTURE

All of the yoga postures are undertaken in the same basic way. Their variations are determined exactly and consistently by the differences in the external shape. The internal dynamic of all yoga postures is always the same. Therein lies the essential simplicity of the yoga method. There are three fundamental principles that apply to the articulation of every posture: the foundation, the core and the dynamic.

THE FOUNDATION

Those parts of the body that are in contact with the floor are actively and evenly engaged against the floor. Grounding the foundation evenly requires that the weight of the body is spread evenly across the entire surface of the foundation. Only when the foundation is evenly grounded can we find the stability that is the root of asana or yoga posture. This does not happen by magic, it requires effort. We must engage the foundation actively into the floor. Not just at the beginning of the posture, but throughout. For the front of the body to be comfortable and stable, the front of the foundation must be actively grounded. Exactly the same is true for the back, left and right.

THE CORE

Whereas the foundation of the posture gives us the possibility of establishing stability (sthira, yoga sutras II. 46), the core of the body gives us the possibility of establishing comfort (sukha, yoga sutras II. 46). The core of the body is the central axis that runs from the perineum to the brain, encompassing the spine and including the throat, tongue, palate, eyes and ears. The key indicators of the quality of the core are the anus, tongue root and eyes. These should always be passive, receptive, easy and comfortable. When the core is able to remain soft then true comfort becomes possible.

THE DYNAMIC

In order for comfortable stability to manifest the infinite beyond duality, yoga postures require a very definite internal dynamic. This dynamic originates in the softness of the core. From there it radiates from the trunk via the limbs into the hands and feet. This unifies the whole body into a single energetic and structural dynamic. When this dynamic is mature it transcends the dualistic distinctions of left and right, top and bottom, front and back, centre and periphery, inside and outside that define our sense of self and other. This dynamic is traditionally known as the bandhas. The bandhas are the heart of every yoga posture.

CONTEXT

These three fundamental principles must occur within the specific context outlined previously. These are the first two limbs of Patanjali's ashtanga yoga: yama and niyama. The principles must, then, be applied sensitively, honestly, openly, directly and generously with a passionate, content commitment to devoted self-enquiry. This weans the mind from its attachment to external sensory stimuli, initiating pratyahara (meditative internalization). This is the fifth limb of ashtanga yoga. It follows naturally from the fourth, pranayama (balancing subtle energies through unhindered breathing). This in its turn occurs within asana, when 'joyful steadiness in the body free from tension manifests the infinite beyond duality'. Pratyahara then deepens into the last three limbs – meditative concentration (dharana), meditative contemplation (dhyana) and meditative absorption (samadhi). The arena and trigger for this process is yoga posture or asana. It is only when the nondual freedom of asana has been established that the nondual release of the breath, and subsequent internalization of the mind can occur. What distinguishes yoga posture from other physical postures is the three principles applied within the context of yama and niyama.

ESTABLISHING YOGA POSTURE

Whether yoga postures are entered from standing, sitting or lying they can all be entered in a number of steps. Each step taken synchronizes exactly with either an inhalation or exhalation. This means that as the inhalation or exhalation begins, the movement of that step begins. As the inhalation or exhalation naturally completes itself, the movement does also. In the beginning you will notice that the body movement is not keeping time with the breath. Stay with the process and slowly but surely it will change. The process of synchronizing body movements with the breath brings a smooth, fluid grace to yoga. It also helps us to safely and effectively establish stability and comfort in a posture step by step, or breath by breath. This integrates the anatomical and physiological bodies. It harmonizes movement and breath. It unifies mind and body. It brings the process and effect of your activities into sharper focus. It creates the space for feedback, and response to that feedback. It allows us to establish a posture safely, from the foundation and the core into the whole body. It teaches us the subtle, consistent dynamic of yoga posture practice.

In the lessons that follow, breath-by-breath instruction is given for learning the postures. Once you have become comfortable in a given posture you can combine steps together. When you do this, remember that there is an underlying principle determining which movements are made on the inhalation, which on the exhalation. If the front of the body is opening relative to the last movement, then you inhale. If it is closing then you exhale. To do otherwise would be to go against the grain of the way the body changes as you breathe.

Equally you can take more steps than those given. You can take a whole breath for or after any or each step to fully accommodate, assimilate and enjoy the purpose of a given step. This will often help in the beginning to clarify exactly what is happening to you. You can also do this as a simple way of slowing your practice, your mind and your self down. This is something that you are free to vary in any way that enriches your practice or deepens your understanding.

The posture instructions are given so that you can make safe and secure step-by-step entry. **Each step is synchronized exactly with an inhalation or an exhalation.** When a step is given in a **bold** typeface it is synchronized with an exhalation. When a step is given in normal typeface it is synchronized with an inhalation. Especially for some of the earlier postures the first few steps are not breath sensitive. However, it is beneficial to become accustomed to activating every step with the breath. In most cases no specific steps are given for leaving a posture. Find your own, comfortable and easy step-by-step way of leaving the postures so that the stability and comfort they have given you comes with you to the next posture.

Even when learning the simple postures in this book great care must be taken. Be sure to follow the instructions given precisely, remembering always to carry over what you learn in one lesson to all those that follow. Be particularly careful with your knees and your neck. They are especially vulnerable, while being crucial to your functioning. Never permit your practice to maintain pain in the knees or neck. There should, in fact, be no discomfort of any kind at all in the neck. In the knee there should never be even a flicker of sensation around the sides and front of the kneecap. Problems can develop in the connective tissue of the knee so incrementally that the damage is done before you recognize any problem or even any pain. Tightness in the back of the knee, however, is not usually a problem. If in doubt, however, consult a qualified professional – preferably one who is knowledgeable about the benefits of yoga.

The hatha yoga postures presented in this book are presented to you in a very definite way. This is designed to allow you to build up your understanding of the hatha yoga method slowly but surely, while at the same time opening your body more and more fully within the context of a comfortable stability. Once the basic concepts of the foundation, softness and the core have been introduced, the subsequent lessons will gradually introduce you to a basic practice format. This format is based on tradition, but it is not a traditional format. It is designed to allow you to progress safely both anatomically and in your understanding. Many of the postures are simplified modifications of the traditional ones. Once you have mastered these modifications the traditional forms will give themselves easily to you.

HOW IT FEELS

Hatha yoga practice is going to make you feel many things. Not all will necessarily be beneficial. Not all will necessarily be enjoyable. Not all those that are beneficial will be enjoyable and not all those that are enjoyable will be beneficial. Through practice based on honest, unprejudiced self-enquiry you will learn which is which.

Resistance: When muscles that are tight from underuse or stress are challenged it can be uncomfortable. This is the natural result of shortened muscles being reopened. It is felt as a dull, surface ache that occurs exactly in tandem with the movement that triggers it. It is not usually sharp, hot, cold, sudden or mind-numbing. This needs to be accommodated, even when the mind tells us to release. No harm will come to you as long as there is no sensation of tearing or pain. By going slowly, methodically into the movement with the foundation stable and activating the dynamic of the bandhas you will soon learn to recognize your limits. Absentmindedness or ambition can dull your sensitivity, causing you to push past your limits without realizing it until suddenly you are confronted with a searing pain.

Pain: This is always a signal that damage is occurring to body tissue. It is not all in the mind. Tissue damage is signalled by pain and results in immediate muscle tightening. This is a protective mechanism that hinders the opening of the muscle you are working on. So, being aggressive and pushing past your limits will not benefit you. By finding your limit daily it will expand, daily. Yoga works through consistent repetition. Not through aggression. Muscles are not bounced. They are elongated slowly, deliberately, from a solid, safe foundation within the spirallic, harmonizing and internalizing dynamic of the bandhas. Then they will not tear.

The edge: Knowing when to stop must be learned. It is a dynamic between body and mind that has many variables. Pain is always unnecessary and unhelpful. Physical resistance is inevitable; mental also. But we must monitor our mental resistance closely. It is a question of finding our edge. This is where any more movement would be aggression and any less would be compromise. A common tendency is to swing between complacent practice and aggressive practice, without ever finding the edge. By going to our edge we challenge the habit of our limitations. We thereby immediately increase our limits, draw on more of our potential. There is a sense of liberation in this, but there can also be a sense of uncertainty as the known is transcended. We have to become familiar and comfortable with this state. Then we have a gauge for going deeper into a posture.

You are going to be introduced to the practice of hatha yoga in 15 lessons. The lessons are presented sequentially so that you learn all that you need as a foundation for any lesson in those that precede it. Therefore, do not miss any lessons out. Even if you are familiar with hatha yoga, you will not be familiar with the approach outlined herein. As you progress through the lessons, the detailed instruction of earlier lessons will be verbally condensed. This allows you to focus on the new points and actions specific to each lesson.

Each lesson has the following parts:

- An introductory image.
- Two or more pages of explanatory text (and pictures where necessary) outlining the relevance of the lesson, what each posture involves, what it teaches and how it relates to the rest of the lessons.
- Detailed instruction of each posture is then given with corresponding illustrations. Each posture has its own double page spread. This allows you to explore the posture without having to turn the page. The left hand page has a colour image of the posture. It also has a brief description of the outline shape and the key points of the posture. The right hand page gives detailed step-by-step instructions with corresponding photographs. Some postures are used in two lessons. This allows you to focus on a particular detail so as to be able to assimilate it before trying to clarify the whole posture.
- At the end of each lesson, a practice sequence is given in the form of small photographs of each of the postures. Some of these postures will be from previous lessons. First go through the postures individually in the sequence they are presented. Take your time to explore the fine details of the postures and experiment so as to clarify the relevance of the instructions. Then put them together dynamically in the single sequence presented visually. This sequence should be repeated daily until the points of the lesson, and the dynamic of its postures has been clarified and embodied.

How long a sequence takes depends on you. On how long you hold the postures and how many repetitions you make – again, this is up to you.

When you have mastered lesson 14 you will know all the postures. The full practice sequence is featured at the end of Lesson 15, along with two shorter sequences – one for strengthening the back, the other for releasing and softening the back (these are useful when you don't have time to do the longer sequences of lesson 13 and 14). Having mastered lesson 14, you will have a wide choice of practice sequences. Each of these can be used according to the time you have available or the emphasis you wish to give to your practice. However, the full practice will give you deeper, more balanced benefits than the others. So try to do the full practice daily. When this is not possible, substitute one of the shorter practice sequences. Ensure, however, that you alternate your choice of shorter practice sequences so that you are not over or under stressing one particular area of your practice.

Take your time. Stay with a lesson until you can do all of the new postures accurately from memory, then move on to the next lesson. This means that you will not be struggling with previous postures as you are learning new ones. Don't be afraid of taking a step or two back through the lessons for clarification. The sequencing of the postures will help you to learn them. If you don't have time for the practice sequence you are on, go back to a shorter earlier one, until you do. The shorter earlier sequences can always be beneficial. Do not think that you will ever be beyond them. The practice sequences of lessons 3 and 4 are particularly beneficial when tired or weak.

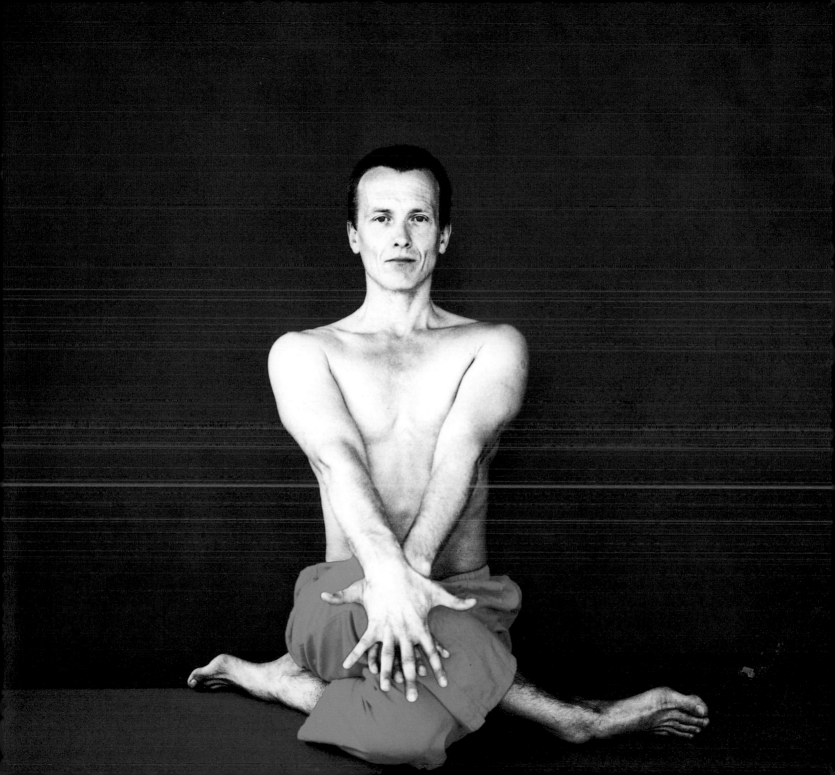

- Yoga is most beneficial if practised regularly. A little often is better than a lot rarely.
- Morning practice sets you up for the day. Evening practice will find you more flexible. Both have their advantages and disadvantages. There is no need to be attached to either.
- Practice on a non-slip surface for sure grip. Practice on an even surface for a stable foundation.
- Never force, push or bounce your way into a posture.
- Indoor practice is preferred as cool external air can be weakening in a strong practice. Never practice in a draught.
- Always practice in a warm place. Cold air on your skin can traumatize muscles that are being heated from within.
- Wear as little as possible – nothing tight, no jewellery. Do you really need a watch?
- If pregnant find a good teacher who is a mother.
- If injured or recovering from injury or illness be sensible, sensitive and patient. Seek competent professional advice.
- Practice on an empty stomach, bowels and bladder. It is disruptive and externalizing to break off your practice to eliminate.
- Do not wipe or towel away sweat. Let it be.
- Stop moving when you need to rest or assimilate but maintain the bandhas and your awareness of your breathing.
- Go slowly after a break, especially after illness.
- Let your practice be a pleasure and a gift, not a whipping stick or a chore.
- Beware of becoming attached to your practice so that you resent other aspects of your life.
- Beware of identifying yourself with your accomplishments or your failures.

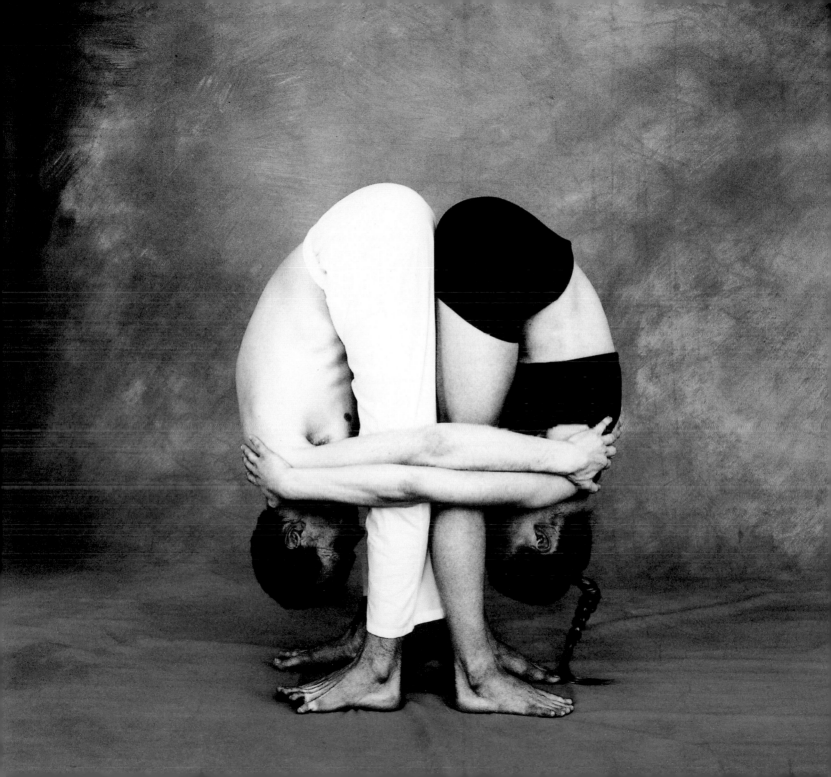

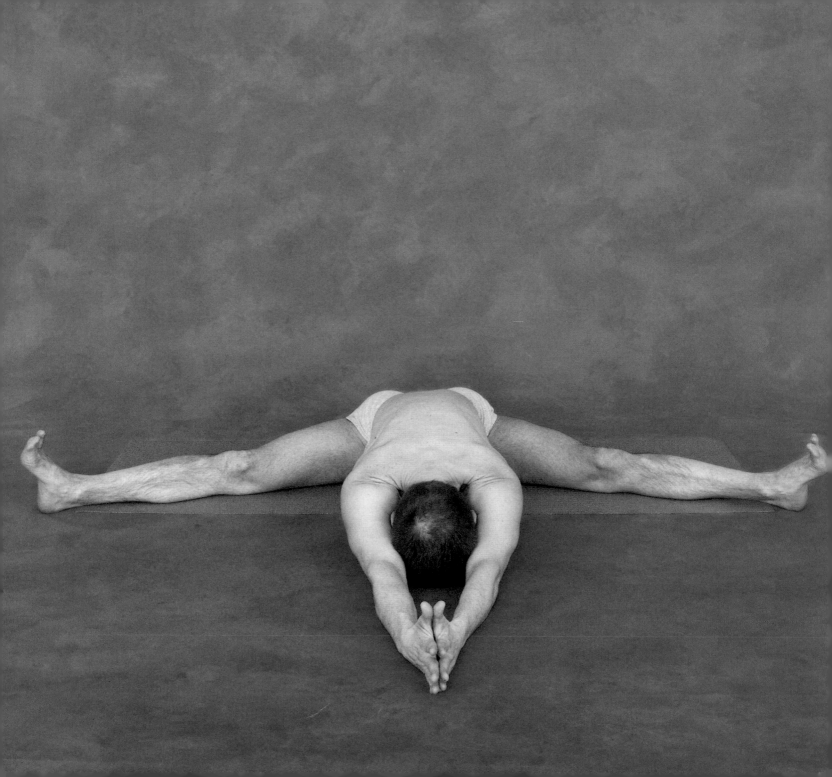

RELAXATION

Hatha yoga is a process of relaxation. Genuine relaxation is a profound state of being wherein there is a complete absence of physical, emotional, mental and spiritual tension. Hatha yoga works systematically through our layers of tension from the most coarse physical level to the most subtle inner dimensions. This begins on the level of the large muscles of the body. It then penetrates into the smaller and deeper, more subtle muscles and body tissues. This includes the vital organs such as liver and kidneys. This is the work of the yoga postures. The process is taken deeper into our emotional structure through yoga breathing or pranayama. It is then taken deeper still, through the mental and to the spiritual level in meditation. As the layers of tension we have accumulated are stripped away we feel, honour and express the fullness of our being more and more freely, more and more fully. We begin to live from inner peace, joy, compassion, wisdom and love. This is not something we have to pretend to. To do so would only generate more tension. It is something that happens by itself as a result of the correct application and contextualisation of the yoga postures. This means to practice them within the guiding context of yama and niyama: sensitivity, honesty, openness, focus, generosity, commitment, contentment, passion, self-reflection and devotion.

Once the muscles of respiration have become more free to move naturally then pranayama (yoga breathing) can begin to occur. Because of the nature of the relationship between breath and emotion this works directly on our emotional field. As new, more open patterns of movement arise in the breath, our old patterns of emotional defence and reaction are undermined. They begin to lose their grip. We are then able to see them for what they are: learned impositions that restrict us from being truly open. In this way they begin to lose their power and eventually atrophy from disuse.

Once the rhythm of the breath has transcended its duality and the distinction between in-breath and out-breath, breathing and not breathing has been rendered insignificant, the dualities of the mind begin to be undermined. The dualities of the mind – that set hot against cold, left against right, black against white, inside against outside, self against other – have been created by the pain of living. This pain creates aversion or dislike. This in turn becomes a barrier separating self from other, us from the world. It is this dualistic perspective that sustains the possibility of our dissatisfaction and disenchantment with life. The purpose of yoga posture and yoga breathing is to free us from this dualism. To allow us to participate freely, fully and directly in the flow of life, as we very much did as infants.

This singular process all begins with learning how to use the yoga postures as tools for relaxation. It is only too easy to use them, unintentionally, as a way of winding ourselves up and generating tension – either through overworking the muscles through aggression, which creates physical tension, or by generating frustration by imposing unrealistic ambition on the actuality of our capability. We must learn to find the internal challenge between action and rest, effort and ease that is a hallmark of the yoga posture dynamic. This is the root of the comfortable quality of yoga posture.

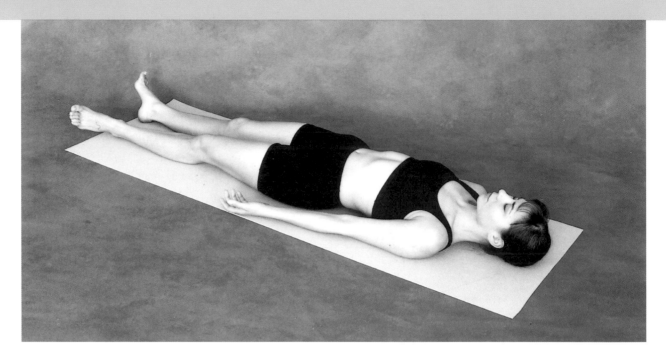

Corpse pose is the most difficult yoga posture – not only in terms of resistance to doing nothing, but also resistance to facing what the stirring effect of our practice brings up. Don't be surprised or discouraged if you experience strong or subtle, continuous or intermittent waves of emotions such as hostility, suspicion, regret, grief, confusion, euphoria, lust, dismay, excitement or anticipation. This is normal and not a sign of faulty practice. Just stay with it. You will then be learning how to meditate. To become able to relax deeply in savasana is much more a mark of accomplishment in hatha yoga than putting a leg behind the head, or doing a handstand. The main difficulty is, of course, the mind. Not having any activity to occupy itself with, it tends to drift away on its habitual patterns of free association by memory. This has to be undermined by paying attention to the sensations of the body relaxing. Rather than using the body's activity as a lattice upon which to weave our awareness, we use its letting go of activity.

Because of the dualistic nature of the analytical mind it is best not to analyse the relaxation process that occurs in savasana. This will block the possibility of accessing a meditative state. Therefore, we take specific account of two body areas only (and then only to begin with). These are the skull and the pelvis. We allow our attention to penetrate the musculature surrounding these areas as fully and deeply as we can. It is here, more than in rest of the body, that deep residual tension lies. As these two areas begin to let go and dissolve into sensations of softening, lengthening, opening and melting, we tune into the inner quality of that process. We allow our attention to be caught in the scent and flavour, the subtle textures, of our letting go. Then we follow that scent as it extends and expands throughout our body, without labelling or categorizing this part of the body and that.

Falling asleep in savasana is permissible. If our practice has broken down some of the armour we have built up to protect us from an ongoing state of tiredness interfering with our daily lives, then we will feel tired. We feel tired because we need to rest and sleep. So, sleep. Don't fight your condition, nurture it and you will nourish and heal yourself. After a while your practice will break down all of the armour, while at the same time teaching you to be more relaxed and sensitive to yourself in the way that you live your life. You will then be able to stay awake and alert during savasana. Daydreaming, however, should not be indulged in. Yoga is first and foremost about presence of mind. You need to be present to your body, and your mind, during the process of letting go.

Because the hatha yoga postures deeply and effectively challenge our emotional body armour, many emotional memories and states can be triggered by your practice. It is especially during savasana, when activity is no longer present to deflect you, that you become aware of these emotions. This can at first be shocking and worrying. However, this is a natural and beneficial process. The tensions, and their underlying trauma, that you have dislodged and released must be resolved. This is only possible if you are willing to invite them freely and fully into your awareness. This is the pragmatic and therapeutic function of both savasana and meditation. As a preliminary training in the meditative process and the hindrances and possibility of surrender, savasana is beyond price. Consequently, it should be done at the end of every session. Beginners should do it before the sitting-in-stillness practice described in lesson 15, while more advanced students should do it after, as a transition to everyday consciousness.

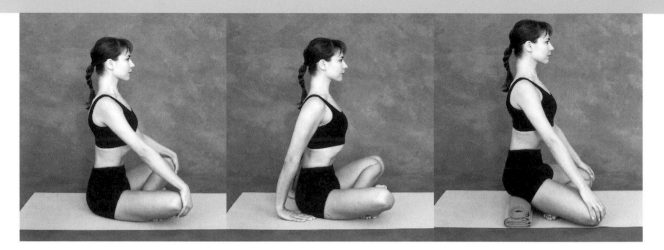

Easy pose is the basic sitting posture. In it we learn how to sit so that the spine can become comfortable and relax. This requires a stable foundation. The foundation of sukasana is the buttock bones, and ankles and feet. Stillness is difficult for most people. Although stillness is the essence of yoga posture and necessary to bring about all of its benefits, most postures do not initially yield enough comfort or stability to permit stillness to occur. Sukasana is therefore a very important, although not very glamorous, posture.

The key to the pose is to separate the knees enough to be able to get onto the front edge of the buttock bones. This allows the sacrum to become vertical and prevents the lower back from collapsing.

If you are too tight in the hips to be able to cross the legs and sit on the front of the buttock bones, you should use some support to lift the buttock bones up so that the knees can more easily separate and go down to be supported by the floor. Alternatively, you can place your hands behind you and use them to keep you on the front edge of the sitting bones.

If the knees stay very high because of tight hips, you can encourage them to relax by supporting them on books, blocks or blankets.

balasana

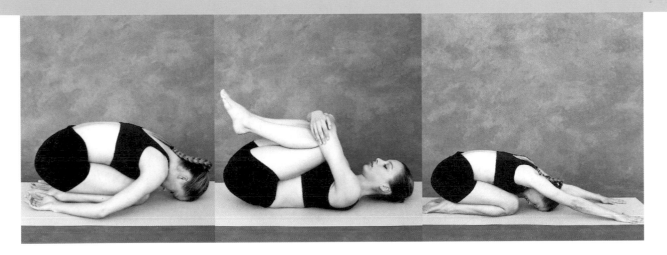

Child pose is a good posture for most people to completely relax in without falling asleep. It permits deep but alert relaxation of the whole body. It also helps to open the back of the lungs and promotes awareness of the back of the body. It can be used at will to rest in-between postures when too tired to work properly or effectively. Remain aware of the natural rhythm of your breath, returning to your practice as soon as it has become stable, fluid and free.

If you are tight in the hips and/or knees and ankles you will find this posture impossible to relax in. You should therefore invert it by lying upside down, with the legs hugged in gently towards the chest and your head on the floor.

Hastabalasana, a more dynamic variation of the child pose, extends the arms forwards and prevents drowsiness when tired.

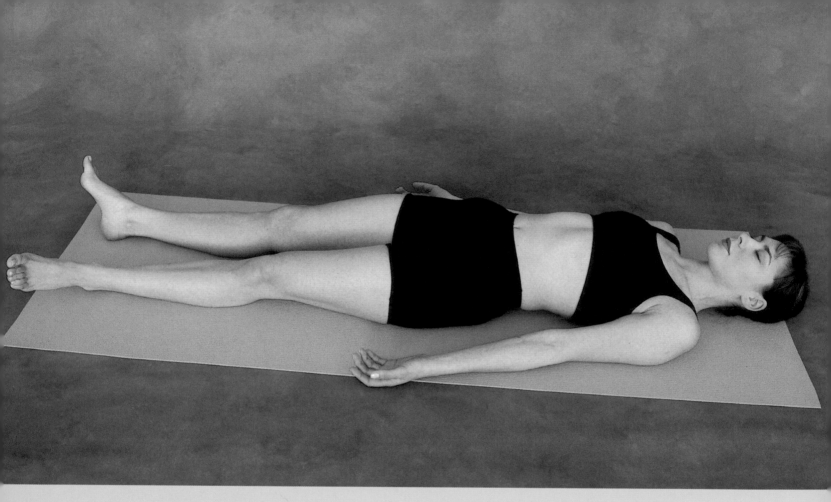

savasana

There is no need for step-by-step breath synchronization in savasana. Make sure that you place your body symmetrically to avoid any discomfort or tension arising from your position. Take special care with the head and neck. Try to centre the head exactly so the neck muscles are even. Make sure that the neck is long with the throat unrestricted. Pay particular attention to releasing the eyes, the perineum and the tongue. Keep your eyes closed until the end. Do not rush. Take your time. Enjoy.

- Lie down on your back.
- Extend your arms alongside you and slightly out to the sides, palms facing upwards.
- Roll your shoulders gently but fully away from your ears, taking the base of your skull away from your shoulders, and lengthening your neck. Make sure you do not overstretch the neck or constrict the throat.
- Lift your pelvis a little off the floor and tuck your buttocks away from you towards your feet, lengthening your lower back gently.
- Straightening your legs, extend them out of the pelvis away from you and completely relax them.
- Place the heels relatively close together, but allow the balls of the feet to roll apart.
- Tuning into the back of your body, adjust yourself as much as possible so that the sameness of feeling on the right and left sides of you, and of each part of your body dissolves any sense of distinction between left and right.
- Take your attention deep inside to the centre of your pelvic floor, and deep into the brain.
- Allow softness to arise in these areas, penetrating them slowly and effortlessly.
- Allow this softness to extend itself in its own time more and more fully, more and more deeply, within you.
- Stay with the changing sensations inside you, feeling whatever there is to feel openly and, if possible, without analysis, evaluation, judgement or reaction.
- Learn through practice to lie comfortably and easily with yourself – the rhythm of your breath, the beating of your heart, the echoes of your pulse – as you slip deeper and deeper into an endlessly opening softness.
- To release the posture, slowly take stock of each part of your body, recognising each part for what it is.
- Then, with your eyes closed, begin to generate movement by first flexing and stretching your fingers and toes, effortlessly and lazily. Without lifting bones against the pull of gravity, allow this movement to extend up the limbs into the pelvis and shoulders, the trunk and spine, the neck and the face.
- Allow your head to roll effortlessly at least once to either side, eyes still closed.
- Roll gently onto your right side, resting your head on your right arm, bringing your left knee up to make you stable and comfortable.
- Eyes still closed, stay as long as you feel like; aware of your breathing, the sensations inside you and the sensations outside of you at the same time.
- Follow the movement of your mind gently and easily, without concern for its direction or content.
- Eventually, keeping your eyes soft, open them without focus to the light.
- Bring your eyes gently to focus, and yourself up to a sitting position.

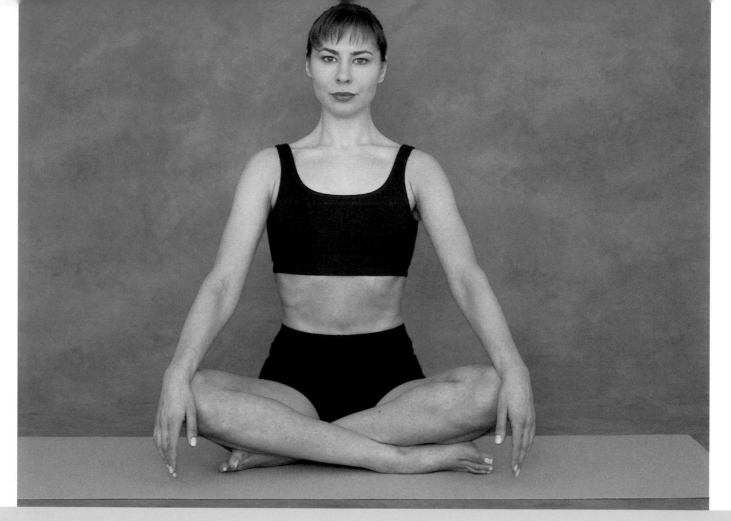

sukasana

This posture is the basic stillness posture. Use something to lift yourself slightly – books, blocks or blankets – if you can't get comfortable directly on the floor. Whatever you use should be firm and with an even surface that does not give under your weight. Sit right on the front edge of your support. Don't neglect this if it is necessary. If you are not yet ready to sit without support you will just create tension, fatigue and discomfort by trying to do without it. Practice of the other postures will soon give you the openness in the hips that you need.

- Sit with your legs relaxed in front of you.
- **Draw your feet in towards your pubic bones and cross your legs.**
- Separate your knees as far as possible until, if possible, the ankles cross. Completely relax your legs. If your legs will not relax, place some firm support underneath each knee so that you can let go deep into the hip socket.
- **Place your hands to the sides of your buttocks.**
- Use your hands to bring yourself forward onto the front edges of your sitting bones (buttock bones).
- **Flatten the palms down into the floor to the sides of your buttocks and, using your arms, lift your trunk upwards, while keeping the pelvis grounded.**
- Lift your head up from the base of the skull, rotating the chin forwards, up and then back. As you move your chin back, roll your shoulders back and, without lifting your pelvis, stretch and lengthen the front of your body from your pubic bone to your chin. This posture is known as easy wheel pose (or chakrasukasana). Hold for ten slow breaths. If this is not comfortable, lengthen the front of the body, with the head looking forward or as far up as you can comfortably take it.
- **Bring your head back to centre and your spine to vertical, while keeping its length and the lift of your chest.**
- Place your hands, wrists or forearms on your knees; hands, arms and shoulders completely relaxed.

Breathing freely, allow your body to relax down into the stability of your pelvis, letting your spine move freely to find its line of effortless elevation out of the pelvis. Consciously release each part of your body patiently and effortlessly, being unconcerned by those areas that don't release.

    If you are dropping and your lower back is rounding, place a book, block or folded rug under your buttock bones, or place your hands behind you and use them and your arms to help keep the spine vertical.

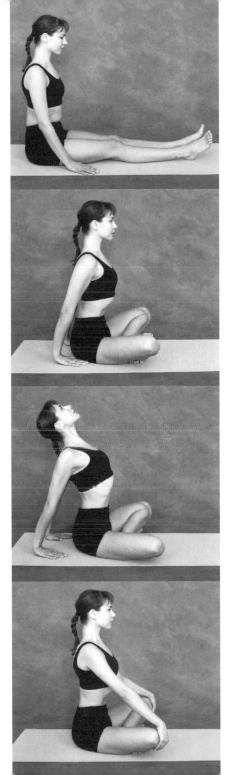

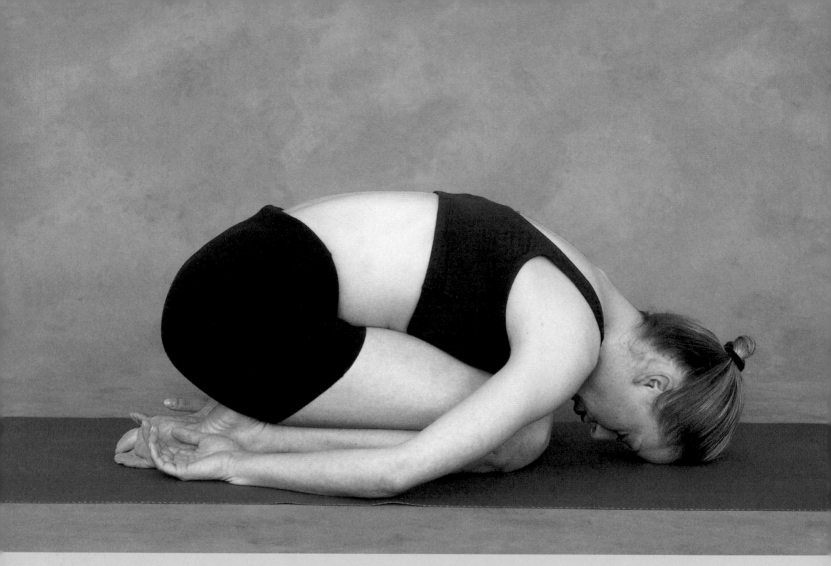

balasana

Keep the body symmetrical, the same contact against the floor with both feet, shins and knees. The same contact between the chest and both thighs, and between the buttocks and both heels. If the posture is uncomfortable due to tightness in the leg joints, invert it by lying on your back and gently hugging your knees into your chest.

- **Kneel, with your buttocks on your heels, feet spread back, legs slightly apart.**
- Lift your weight off your heels and extend your arms and hands forwards until your hands reach the floor.
- **Place your knees and feet hip-width apart, joining the edges of the big toes together.**
- Pushing back with your hands, bring your buttocks gently down onto your heels so that you have the same contact between each buttock and its heel.
- **Drop your chest slowly down onto your thighs so that you have the same contact between each thigh and its side of the chest.**
- Bring your arms back alongside you and place the backs of your hands on the floor by the feet.
- **Relax the whole body so that you sink down more deeply onto your thighs and heels.**
- Allow the back of your body to open, broaden and expand as you breathe in.

If this posture is uncomfortable, then lie on your back with your head on the floor and hug your knees gently in towards your chest.

Hold the posture – feeling relaxation spreading through your body down into the floor. Consciously release each part of your body patiently and effortlessly, being unconcerned by those areas that don't release. Maintain a clear awareness of the flow of your breath lengthening and deepening spontaneously. Feel each exhalation beginning and ending freely and fully. Come to a sitting position when ready.

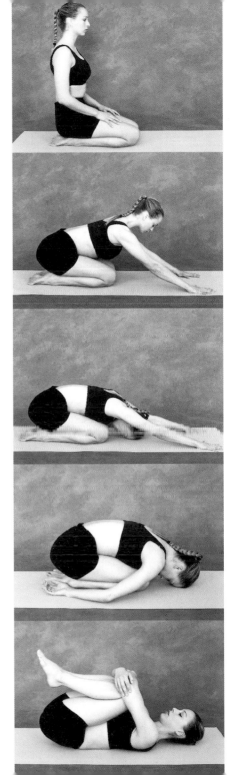

THE RELAXATION PRACTICE

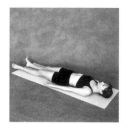 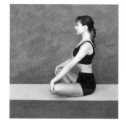 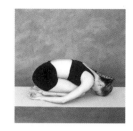 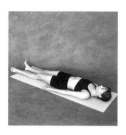

savasana p22   sukasana p24   balasana p26   savasana p22

This practice can be used for a short relaxation or rejuvenation practice – hold balasana and sukasana 100 slow breaths minimum, hold savasana as required without counting or timing.

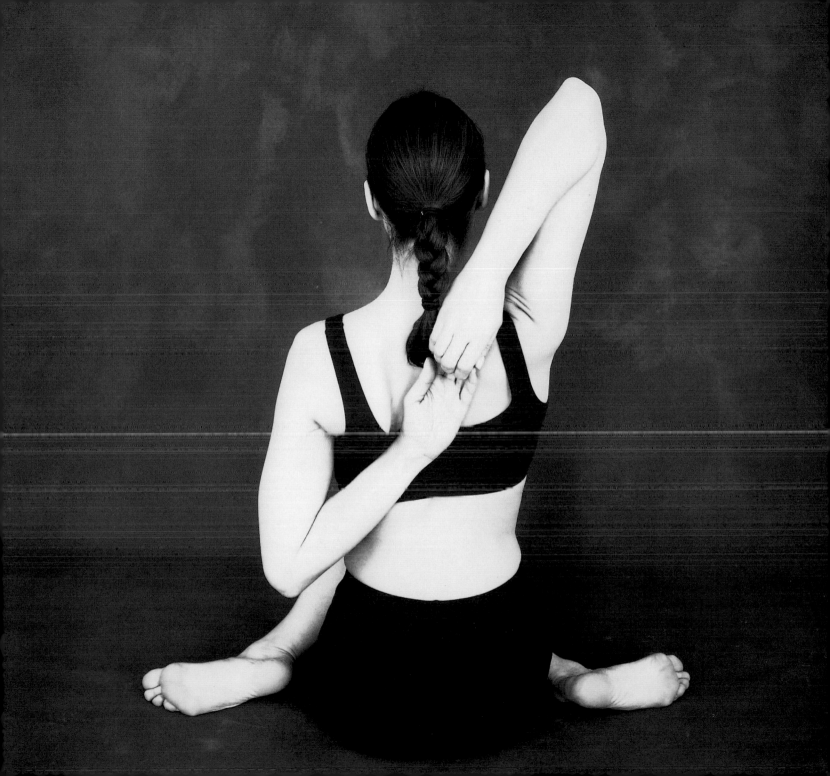

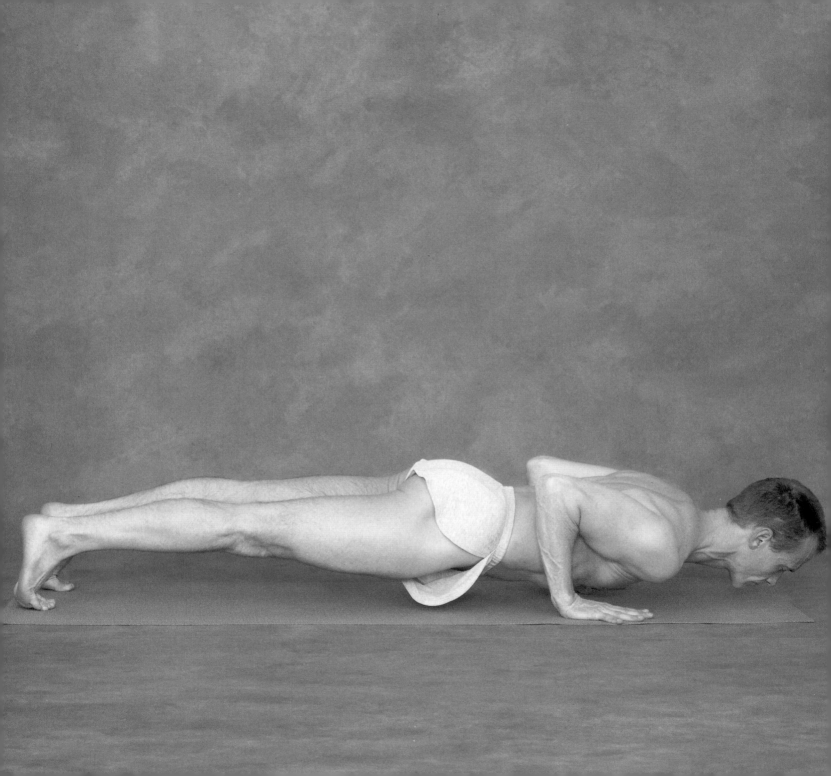

THE FOUNDATION

The foundation determines the quality and impact of all yoga postures: just the same as in any building, where distortions or inaccuracies in the foundations will be reflected throughout the whole structure. Therefore concern for the quality of the foundation is paramount and perpetual. The foundation is all those parts of the body that make contact with the floor. They make contact with the floor actively and evenly. That means that they share the weight of the body equally across their total surface area. It also means that they engage the floor actively. There is a definite pushing downwards. This is not aggressive. It is firm, stable and continuous. This makes the foundation alive, sensitive and responsive. This in turn makes it more possible and likely that the rest of the body will be also.

When the foundation is the feet, body weight is distributed evenly between them, between the balls of the feet and the heels and between the inner and outer edges of the feet. This means that the four corners of the feet are dynamically and equally grounded – the balls of the big and little toes and the inner and outer heels. When the foundation is one foot, the same principles and process apply.

When the foundation is only the hands the principle is exactly the same. Body weight is distributed evenly between the two hands, between the bases of the fingers and the heels of the hands, and between both sides of each hand. When the foundation is the hands and the feet, or one hand and one foot, the principles and process remain the same. This consistency covers all the postures, without exception. Only when the foundation is evenly grounded can the spine and lungs be balanced and stable. No matter whether we are vertical or horizontal, upright or inverted, sitting or squatting. Even and stable support for the spine and lungs depends on an even and active foundation. This gives us the stability that is the root of asana or yoga posture.

Our first concern in any posture is to be clear about what the foundation is. If we put anything else on the floor the posture will be distorted and not deliver its potential. It may even result in injury. This is especially likely in inverted postures. If we place ourselves incorrectly in the shoulderstand and its variations we may put pressure on the vertebrae that causes discomfort and even injury. Of course it may be that we do not have the capacity to avoid this. So we must be honest, open and generous to ourselves by not imposing our ambitions on our limitations. Instead we must go back and develop our capacity in other accessible postures.

When we know what the foundation is then we can use it to support the rest of the body evenly and easily, giving us the possibility of comfortable stability.

In this lesson we will focus on the use of the foundation in standing, sitting, kneeling and upside down postures. The principles you will learn with these postures can then easily be applied to other postures. The foundation necessary for face-down postures will be clarified in lesson 13 for strengthening the back.

trikonasana

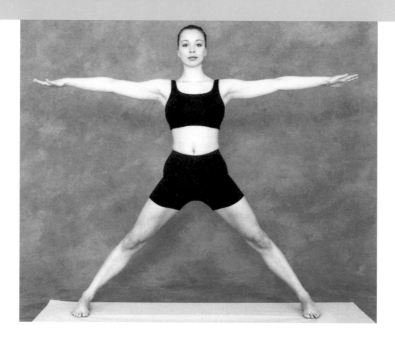

Triangle pose teaches you how to ground the feet. Only when they are grounded can they give us the support we need. This requires a specific muscular action in the legs, especially the thighs. Normally we use our muscles to move our bones through space. In a yoga posture we use our muscles to prevent us from moving through space. We must, therefore, use them differently. Rather than pulling on the bones by activating a strong contraction in the centre of the muscle belly, we want to cradle the bone. We want to wrap the muscles tightly round the bone to support them and make them stable. We can then become comfortable enough to sustain the posture and allow it to do its work of freeing a given part of our body from tension. We must learn to re-educate the muscles.

This involves learning to work them deliberately, specifically and gently. Too much muscular effort will create too much central contraction. It will also tire the muscles and bring on instability and fatigue. We need to create a gentle, sustainable peripheral contraction at the origin and insertion (each end) of the muscles. The main effort is directed toward creating resistance to work against in the feet, by pressing them down firmly into the floor. Luckily it is not necessary to know any anatomy to do this, it is simply a question of feeling. We must only become able to distinguish between muscles tightening away from the bone and muscles wrapping in towards it. This is mostly a matter of practice. If you quickly start to shake or tire, ease up a little and find another way to use your thigh muscles.

In effect, what you are bringing about is a suction inwards of bulk of the muscles in the thigh. The feeling you are looking for is one of sucking into the bone – as if the bone itself were sucking the muscle tissues into itself for safety and comfort. This can be done and felt as a single process encompassing the length of the thigh muscles in the front, back and insides of both thighs. As your practice develops you will become more and more aware of this process and more and more able to refine and stabilize it. In the beginning, however, your muscles will keep losing their grip. Often you won't even notice. When you do, just reassert the sucking action so that it feels as if the muscles are becoming the bone.

Until you have mastered this process you run the risk of overworking muscles such as the hamstrings or those of the lower back. Therefore it is important that you proceed with caution and patience. Do not hold postures for too long until you have mastered this peripheral muscular contraction. Neither should you force your body to extremes of movement – even those you are well capable of. If you do not have a stable, secure foundation you are not safe. When the thighs are working correctly, the muscles seal into the bone, the kneecaps are lifted up towards the thighs and into the knee joint, while the back of the knee joint opens out. When the action is even all round the thigh, then the knee will be centred and much less vulnerable.

When this peripheral muscular contraction is possible in the thighs, you will be able to fully ground your feet. Even before then, you can use the feet to ground themselves as much as possible. This, in turn, will give you feedback to facilitate using the thighs correctly. It will also automatically engage the muscles of the calf and shin, sucking them into the shinbone. When the foot is not worked correctly, the lower leg cannot fully support the bones of the skeleton as a whole. To ground your feet, spread your weight evenly between the left foot and the right, between the heels and the balls of the feet, and between the inner and outer edges of the feet. Now press down firmly and evenly with the four corners of each foot – the ball of the big toe, the ball of the little toe, the inner heel and the outer heel.

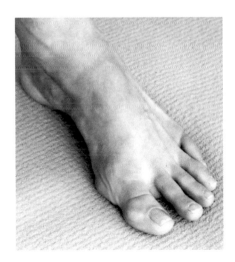

dandasana

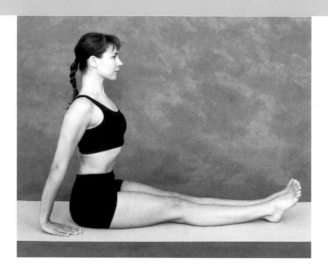

Staff pose teaches you how to use the legs in exactly the same way as trikonasana, but without having the floor to resist against. This is a little more tricky, but just as important. Again it is a matter of activating peripheral muscular contraction. This means keeping the central muscle belly passive as you suck the muscles of the thighs into the bone, while pressing the heels and knees down so the hamstrings engage. Dandasana is the basis of many seated postures: extensions, twists and forward bends in particular. In order for these postures to be effective and safe, the technique of dandasana must be mastered and applied to them. Dandasana also teaches the correct sitting position for the buttock bones. In hatha yoga we almost always sit to the front edge of the buttock bones. This keeps the sacrum more vertical, the hipbones just in front of the buttock bones and prevents the lower back from collapsing. This is especially important for the postures in lessons 10 and 11. If these postures are done from the back of the buttock bones the spine will not be able to release, soften, lengthen or strengthen.

Dandasana also teaches how to use the hands when they are a part of the foundation. This is based on exact placing of the hands. There should be a small, equal space between all the fingers, with a little more separating the thumb from the index finger. The fingers should be extending along the floor, with the heel of the hand and the bases of the fingers pressing firmly into the floor. Because of the large mound at the base of the thumb the base of the index finger tends to lift off the floor. When this happens, the muscles of the inner arm are not properly supported and the outer arm muscles compensate for this by overworking. They then tire easily, and can, in the long run, become overdeveloped. This can then create difficulties in opening the shoulders, doing backbends and doing inversions.

Dandasana also teaches the correct use of the feet when they are *not* part of the foundation. This involves using the feet to express and support the dynamic of the bandhas. By using the feet correctly, the lower leg muscles of the calf and shin are properly engaged, sucking into the shinbone. When the foot is not worked correctly, the leg cannot be fully engaged. The ball of the foot should be broad, with the toes lengthening upwards without straining the tendons. The front ankle is open, soft and long without shortening the Achilles tendon, while the Achilles tendon itself is long without shortening and tightening the front ankle. The inner ankle is extended so that the inner and outer edges of the feet are both the same distance from the head of the thighbone. This will be focused on more fully in lesson 4.

The grounding action of the foundation (legs, buttock bones and hands) in dandasana clearly demonstrates the indivisibility of the body in action. If the foundation is correctly engaged, the spine lifts and lengthens, the lungs have more room, the breath becomes more free.

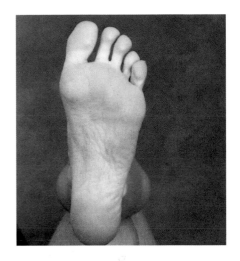

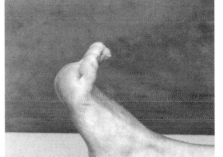

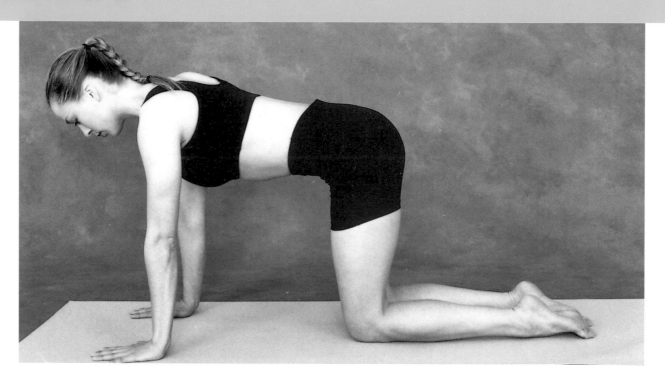

Dog pose   teaches you how to use the hands when they are a major part of the foundation, especially how to work back from them to the rest of the foundation. It is a very simple posture, but is very important as its hand action forms the basis of the other dog poses, upwards-dog and downwards-dog, as well as other postures that are crucial to the dynamic aspect of traditional practice. It is important to get the line of the arms and thighs correct. They must be vertical – shoulders above wrists, hips above knees.

ardapindasana

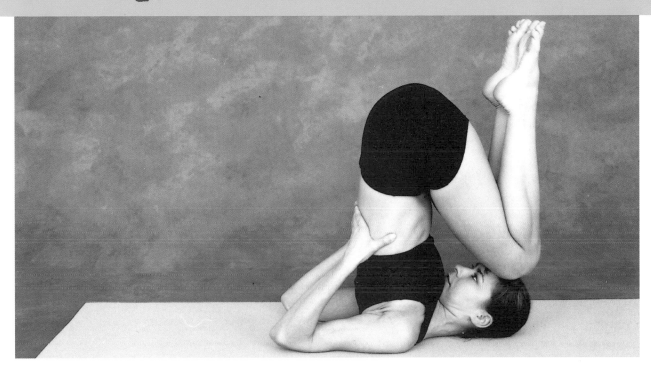

Embryo pose teaches how to lie safely on the shoulders with the support of the elbows and upper arms. This is crucial to all of the variations of the shoulderstand that constitute the kernel of the rejuvenation aspect of the practice. The larger vertebrae where the back becomes the neck are especially vulnerable to irritation in these inversions – but only when they are not applied correctly. Learning to support the shoulders with the elbows and upper arms is crucial for the shoulderstand and plough poses. Many people hurt and injure themselves when trying these postures. This is not because the postures are dangerous, but because the student is ignorant of the correct technique or unready for the postures. Both the shoulderstand and the headstand are advanced postures. Until the body has been well trained in the internal dynamic of yoga posturing, and especially in how to resist the effect of gravity in each part of the body individually, these two postures are not safe. The beauty of a step-by-step approach to yoga is that all postures become almost effortlessly accessible when properly prepared for by prior, simpler postures that teach the internal dynamic required in a safer, easier context.

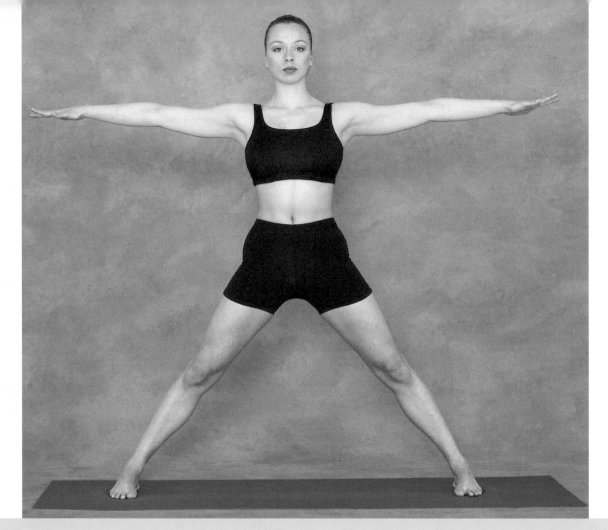

trikonasana

This posture is the basic standing posture. The legs are spread wide with the feet parallel to each other. The feet are grounded and alive, the legs strong. The weight of the body is spread evenly between the feet, between the heels and the balls of the feet and between the inner and outer edges of the feet. The arms are parallel to the floor. The trunk is upright and relaxed. Look straight ahead. Focus on the dynamic of the feet and legs and the broadening they give to the pelvis, the lift they give to the trunk.

- Stand with your legs spread wide apart, hands on your hips. This posture is hastatrikonasana.
- **Make your feet parallel. Judge this by the space between the first two toes.**
- Spread your body weight evenly between the left and right foot.
- **Spread your body weight evenly between the heels and the balls of your feet.**
- Spread your body weight evenly between the inner and outer edges of your feet.
- **Suck the thigh muscles into your thighbones so that your legs become straight and strong but not tense. The kneecaps will lift, the backs of the knees open. Do not hyperextend into the back of the knee.**
- Check that your body weight is still even across the surface of the feet.
- **Broaden the ball of the foot, pressing out from the ball of the big toe to the ball of the little toe.**
- Lengthen the inner edge of the foot, pressing back from the ball of the big toe to the inner heel so that the inner ankle is taken back.
- **Lengthen the outer edge of the foot, pressing back from the ball of the little toe to the outer heel. Connect this action to the broadening of the ball of the foot.**
- Broaden the heels, pressing from the inner heel to the outer heel in a rotating motion, while keeping both feet firmly grounded.
- **Ground the four corners of each foot – ball of the big toe, ball of the little toe, inner heel and outer heel – evenly and fully.**
- Extend the arms parallel to the floor and raise the chest. Keep the shoulders relaxed and look ahead, keeping the feet alive and the legs strong.

Hold the posture – with awareness of the flow of your breath – until ready to release. Release by bringing the feet together on an exhalation.

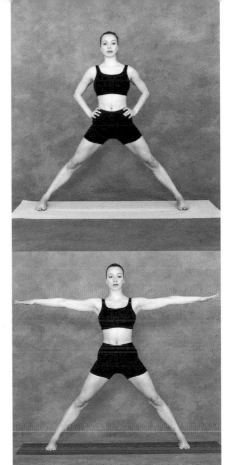

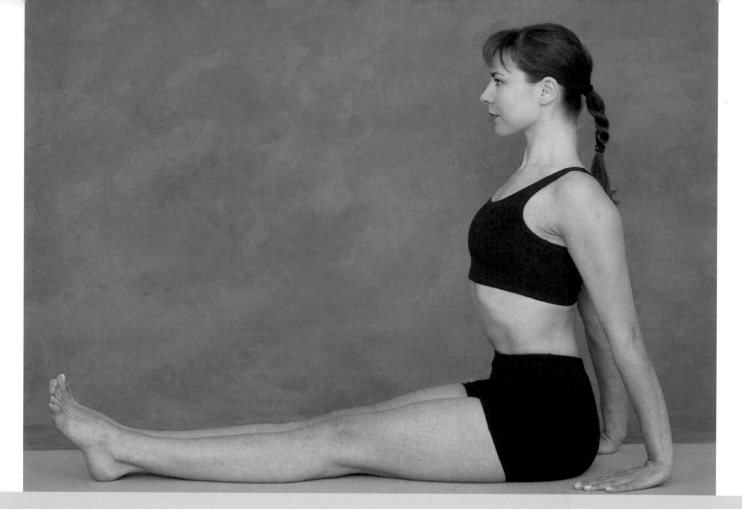

dandasana

This posture is the basic sitting posture. The legs are extended in front of you and are active. The heels and knees are pressing down, while the thigh muscles are being sucked into the bone. The feet touch at the balls of the big toes and inner ankles. They are active, with the balls of the feet broad, and the front ankle, inner ankle and Achilles tendon long. The trunk is vertical, arms supporting the extension, chest open. The hands are part of the foundation – use them. The weight is evenly distributed from the heels to the hands, including the buttock bones. Look straight ahead. Focus on grounding the legs and hands, and feeling the lift that gives to the trunk without disturbing the pelvis.

- Sit with your legs relaxed in front of you.
- **Make sure that the hips are aligned and bring your inner heels together with legs still relaxed.**
- Bring the balls of the big toes and the inner anklebones in contact with each other, so that the inner and outer edges of the feet are the same distance away from you.
- **Suck the thigh muscles into the thighbones so that the kneecaps are pulled up and in, the knee bones go down and the shin and thigh bones line up.**
- Broaden the balls of your feet, allowing the centre of each to lead away from your ankle and not the ball of the big toe.
- **Lengthen the front ankle, Achilles tendon and inner ankle so the inner ankles engage against each other firmly.**
- Place your hands by your buttocks, fingers pointing towards the feet, and use your hands to bring you to the front edge of your buttock bones.
- **Press down into the floor with the bases of your fingers and the heels of your hands so that the trunk lifts and the spine lengthens. Do not lift the buttock bones.**
- Lifting your armpits, relax your shoulders down, allowing your shoulder blades to drop down your back.
- **Clarify the sucking action of your legs and the dynamic of your feet.**

Hold the posture – with awareness of the flow of your breath – until ready to release.

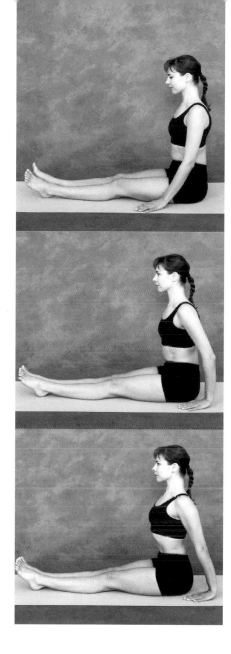

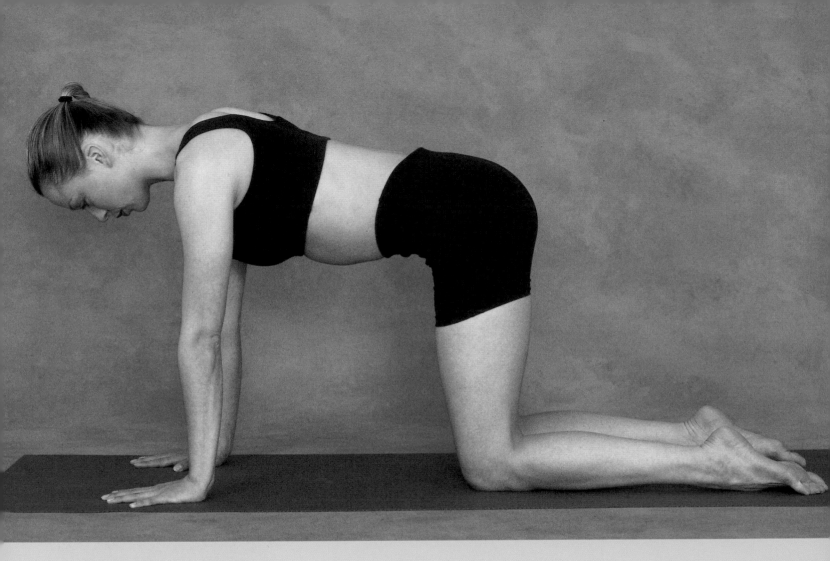

svanasana

This posture is known colloquially as the all-fours pose. However, there are more accurately six points of contact with the floor – the hands, the knees and the feet. The arms and thighs are vertical, the shoulders are directly above the wrists, the hips directly above the knees. The feet can be tucked in or the toes extended back. The shoulders should be relaxed. The weight is even between the hands and legs.

- **Kneel with your buttocks on your heels, feet spread back, legs slightly apart.**
- Lift your weight off your heels and extend your arms and hands forwards until your hands reach the floor.
- **Walk your hands forwards until they are under the shoulders.**
- Bring your weight forwards so that the thighs are vertical.
- **Relax your body and press down firmly and evenly with your hands. Lengthen your fingers and press firmly with the heels of the hands and the bases of the fingers, especially the index finger.**
- Check the line of your arms and thighs, making sure you have not brought your weight too far forwards.
- **Make sure your body weight is spread evenly on your foundation.**

Hold the posture – with awareness of the flow of your breath – until ready to release. Release back to a kneeling position.

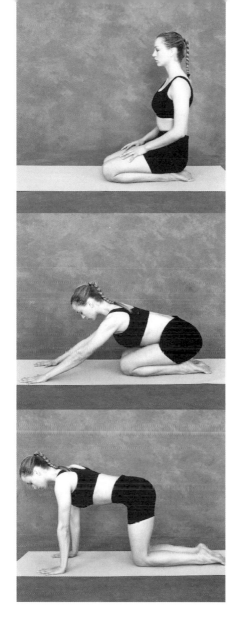

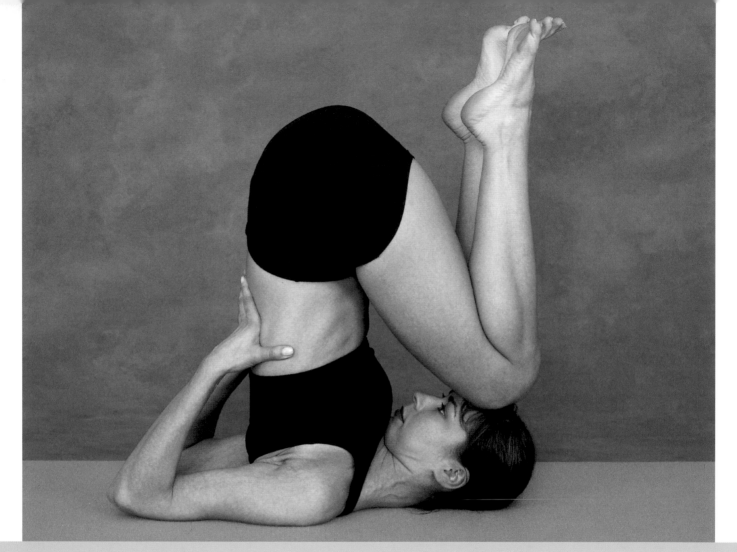

ardapindasana

This posture is the basic inverted posture. The weight is spread evenly between the shoulders, elbows and upper arms. As little weight as possible is carried on the vertebrae. The shoulders are kept away from the ears to keep the neck long and free. This should be a restful posture. The back will only be straight for those with long thighs, so allow your back to round so that the knees comfortably reach the forehead.

- Lie comfortably on your back, arms and legs outstretched, shoulders away from your ears.
- **Bend your legs and draw your feet close into your buttocks, knees together.**
- Extending your arms past your buttocks, press your palms firmly into the floor.
- **Pushing with your hands, roll your knees up towards your chest so your buttocks and lower back rise away from the floor.**
- Bring your hands up to support your back, while lowering your knees onto your forehead.
- **Draw your feet back towards the buttocks, bringing your heels as close to them as you can.**

Hold the posture – with awareness of the flow of your breath – until ready to release. Release by reversing the steps you used to enter (without necessarily synchronizing with your breath).

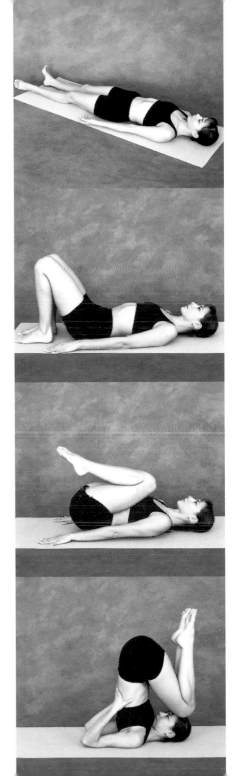

THE FOUNDATION PRACTICE

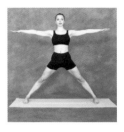

trikonasana p38

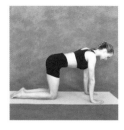

svanasana p42

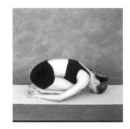

balasana p26

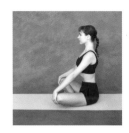

sukasana p24

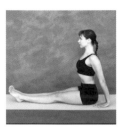

dandasana p40

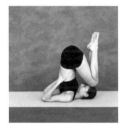

ardapindasana p44

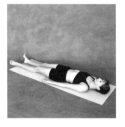

savasana p22

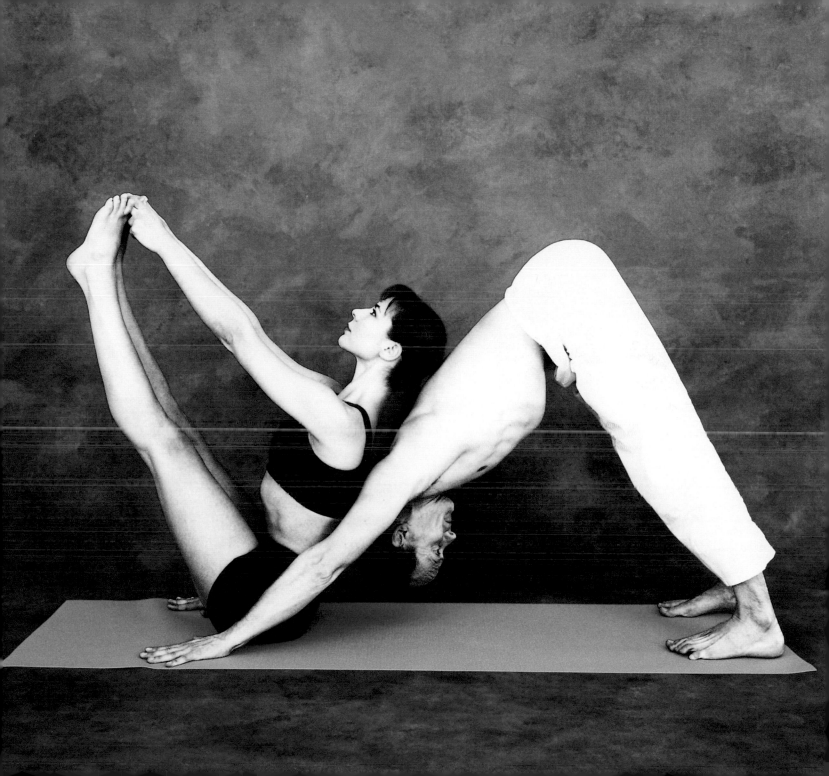

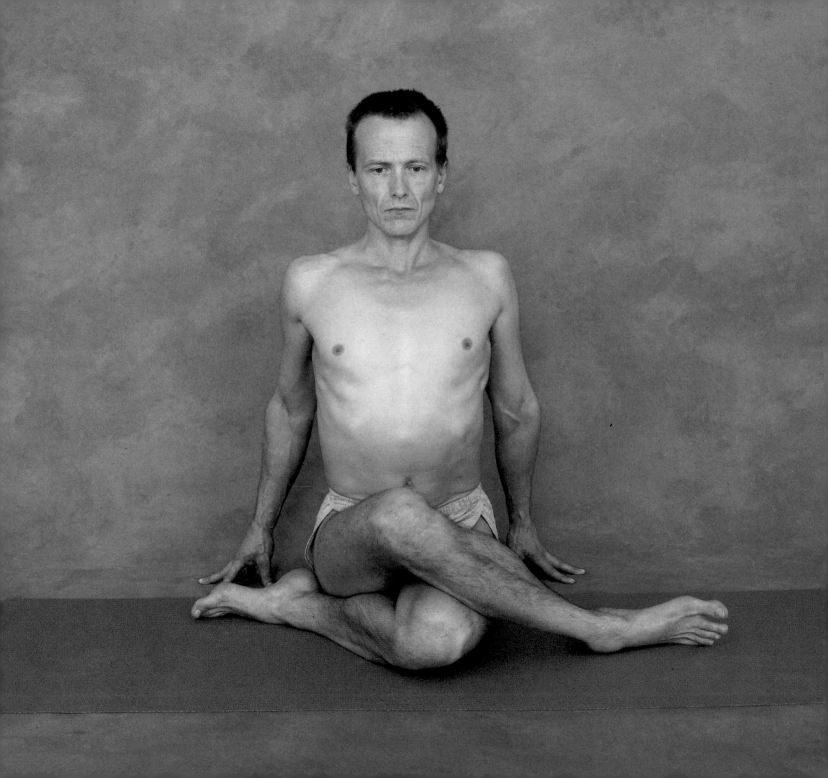

THE CORE

The core of your body is the core of your yoga practice. Its quality determines the quality not only of your posture, but your breathing also. The quality of your core, then, determines the quality and effect of your practice. Your core is the central axis of your body, running down from the brain, through the throat and spinal cord and into the pelvic floor. In effect it encompasses the muscles of the ears, eyes, mouth and face, the solar plexus, navel and anus. This axis is vital to our wellbeing. Yoga is a journey back to our true nature. It is a journey of giving up, of letting go, of surrender of all that which is only momentary. Yoga confronts us with the physical, emotional and mental patterns of restriction within which we have bound and identified ourselves. This confrontation must occur within the context of sensitive, honest, open, direct, generous, passionate, committed and devoted self-enquiry. Then it will bring us to freedom in our core.

The quality of our core is the root of the 'comfortability' of a yoga posture. The softer and more open our core, the more any yoga posture can be comfortable and enhance and express a joyful ease. Likewise, the more comfortable our posture and open our core, the more freely, effortlessly and easily we breathe. The core then is the root of both posture and breathing. To enhance and refine them, we must soften and release our core. This relationship works both ways. The tension in our outer bodies expresses tension in our core. As we release this outer tension, we release our core and initiate a self-perpetuating cycle of release. There is one vital and indispensable factor upon which this cycle depends: awareness. We cannot force our core to give up its deep tension. We can only undermine it by practising the yoga postures from awareness of the quality of our core. Very often, especially when being physically, emotionally or mentally challenged, we tighten our core to give us resilience and power. This habit is counterproductive to yoga. To undermine it we must learn to remain in contact with our core so that we can keep it as soft and open as we can. In the beginning this may be limited, but as our practice progresses it becomes less and less so. Awareness of the quality of our core, then, becomes the kernel of our practice.

The root of this awareness lies in the pelvic floor. We must learn to be constantly aware of the quality of the perineum and anus. They should always be soft, passive and yielding. The apex of this awareness is in the mouth. The jaw, palate and tongue should always be soft, passive and yielding. We can use the anus and tongue root as the essential indicators of the quality of our core. We try to breathe, feel, move and practice from a continuous awareness of the quality of these areas. If we find tightness or tension developing in either one we try to release it. First, see if they soften by holding your attention on them. If this does not work, stabilize and secure your foundation, then make sure that the rest of your body is involved in expressing the singular dynamic of the bandhas. If none of these reminders work, back off a little. You may be asking too much of yourself, and the resistance you are feeling is healthy and normal.

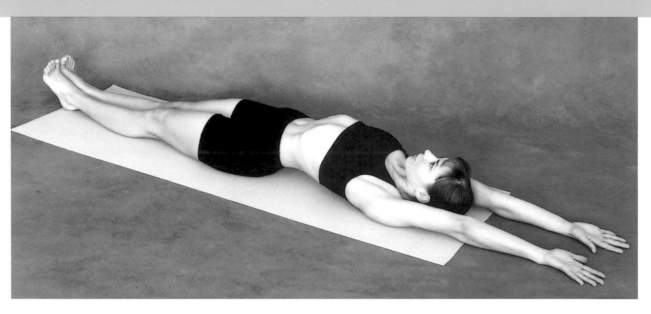

Stretching pose teaches how to lengthen the trunk, spine and core. It facilities awareness of the core, and stimulates deeper breathing without imposing on the respiratory muscles. The trunk is emphasized by extending the arms alongside the ears. This simple dynamic in the outer body harnesses awareness and allows us to focus on the quality of the core. As we raise the arms we can feel the trunk, the spine, and therefore the core, lengthening. It activates the whole body without challenging any muscular restrictions.

suptabadakonasana

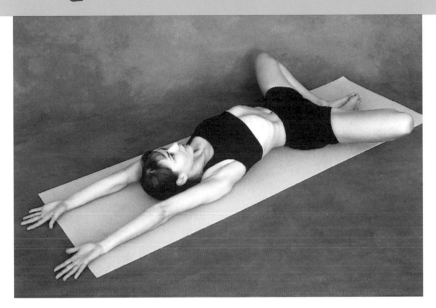

Reclining cobbler also teaches us how to lengthen the trunk, spine and core; and how to elongate and emphasize the trunk by extending the arms alongside the ears. It stimulates deeper breathing without imposing on the respiratory muscles, and is especially useful for tuning into the pelvic floor and learning how to isolate the various muscle groups found there. The positioning of the feet also stretches the pelvic floor, facilitating sensitivity to the state and quality of the pelvic floor. Reclining cobbler helps to clarify the musculature of the pelvic floor by stretching it. It helps enormously in your practice if you are able to identify and isolate three sets of muscles in the pelvic floor: the anal muscles at the back near to the coccyx, the uro-genital muscles at the front near the pubis, and the perineal muscles in between.

Women, especially mothers, seem to have a greater facility for exploring and relating to the pelvic floor. Nevertheless, both genders benefit from greater control of these muscles, mainly because it is important to keep them passive in your practice. To be able to be sure that they are passive, it helps to know what it feels like when they are active. The fact is that most of us are tight-arsed. This may originate in potty training, but is constantly reinforced by life, and even by poor yoga practice. Reclining cobbler can be used to learn to pacify the whole pelvic floor, and to distinguish actively between all of the muscles. You can explore them during the posture by alternately contracting the muscles of the pelvic floor as a whole, and separately. Find your own rhythms and patterns of contraction and release, so that you develop a deep and clear awareness and control of all the pelvic floor muscles.

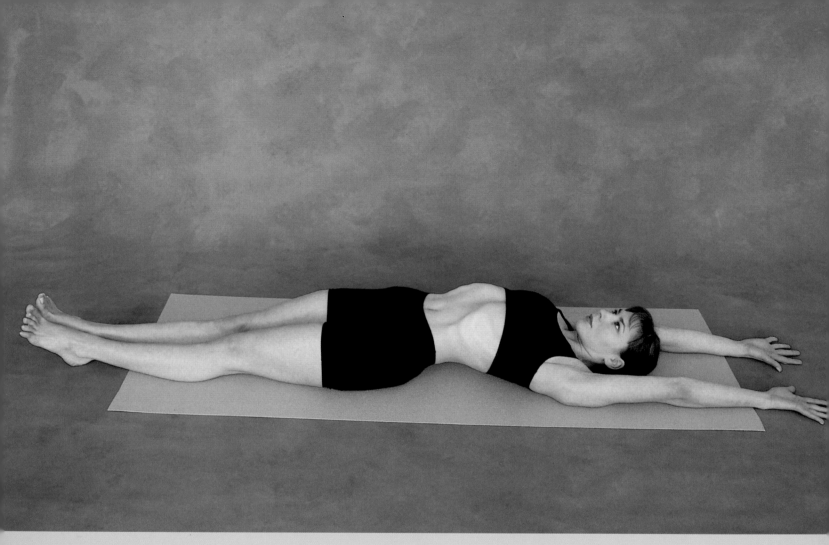

suptahastasana

This posture is easily accessible to everyone. Keep the body symmetrical and the lower back soft. Keep the balls of the feet broad, the front and inner ankles long, and the toes long. Suck the thigh muscles into the bone as you press the heels and knees down. Keep the shoulders relaxed and away from the ears, and the arms and hands engaged. Focus on the length in your abdomen and the impact that has on your chest and breathing, while making sure your core is soft.

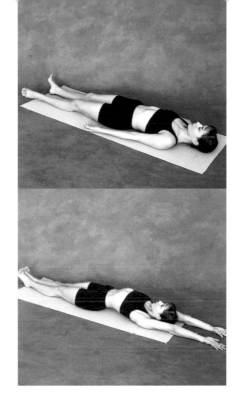

- Lie down on your back and extend your arms alongside you and slightly out to the sides.
- **Roll your shoulders gently but fully away from your ears, lengthening your neck. Make sure you do not overstretch the neck or constrict the throat.**
- Lift your pelvis a little off the floor and tuck your buttocks away from you towards your feet, lengthening your lower back gently.
- **Straightening your legs, extend them out of the pelvis away from you. Press the inner edges of the feet together with contact between the balls of the big toes and inner ankles, and make the legs strong by sucking the thigh muscles into the bone.**
- Take your attention deep into your pelvic floor, and deep into the brain and face, allowing them both to soften and open. Be especially aware of your anus, tongue, eyes and ears releasing.
- **Making the fingers long and the palms broad, lengthen and straighten your arms.**
- Keeping your legs strong and straight, your feet pressing together, raise your arms up off the floor in an arc, extending them alongside your ears, hands shoulder-width apart.
- **Press the backs of your hands down into the floor and lengthen your arms out of your armpits, keeping them straight and strong, palms broad and fingers long.**
- Keeping your arms dynamically extended, lengthen your trunk, spine and core by taking your ribcage along the floor away from your pelvis, maximizing the distance between the breastbone and the pubic bone and between the armpits and the hipbones.

Hold the posture – maintaining a clear and continuous awareness of your core (especially the anus and the tongue so they remain soft and passive), be aware of the free flow of inhalation and exhalation as you keep the arms and legs dynamically charged – until ready to release. Release into savasana.

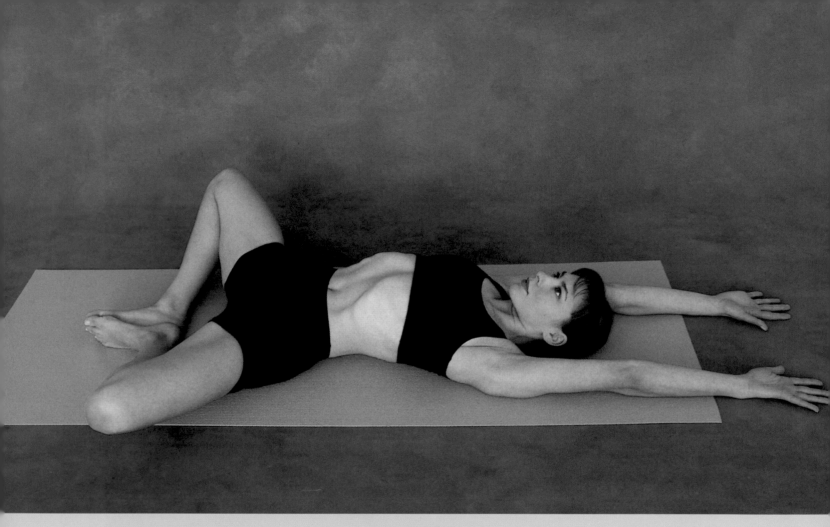

suptabadakonasana

Keep the body symmetrical, the lower back soft. Keep the shoulders relaxed and away from the ears, and keep the arms and hands engaged. If you can not comfortably press the soles of the feet together, then cross the ankles. In either case, make sure that there is not subliminal tension or gripping in the thighs or hips sockets. Let the legs relax – the pressing action comes from the feet and should stimulate release in the hips. Focus on the length in your abdomen and the impact that has on your chest and breathing, while making sure your core is soft.

- Lie down on your back and extend your arms alongside you and slightly out to the sides.
- **Roll your shoulders gently but fully away from your ears, lengthening your neck. Make sure you do not overstretch the neck or constrict the throat.**
- Lift your pelvis a little off the floor and tuck your buttocks away from you towards your feet, lengthening your lower back gently.
- **Bending your legs, bring the soles of your feet together and press the heels and balls of the feet together.** If this is not comfortable or possible, simply cross your ankles.
- Take your attention deep into your pelvic floor, and deep into the brain and face, allowing them both to soften and open. Be especially aware of your anus, tongue, eyes and ears releasing.
- **Making the fingers long and the palms broad, lengthen and straighten your arms.**
- Pressing your feet together, raise your arms up off the floor in an arc, extending them alongside your ears, the hands shoulder-width apart.
- **Press the backs of your hands down into the floor and lengthen your arms out of your armpits, keeping them straight and strong, palms broad and fingers long.**
- Keeping your arms dynamically extended, lengthen your trunk, spine and core by taking your ribcage along the floor away from your pelvis, maximizing the distance between the breastbone and the pubic bone and between the armpits and the hipbones.

Hold the posture – maintaining a clear and continuous awareness of your core (especially the anus and the tongue so they remain soft and passive), be aware of the free flow of inhalation and exhalation as you keep the arms dynamically charged, and the feet pressing if they are together – until ready to release. Release into savasana.

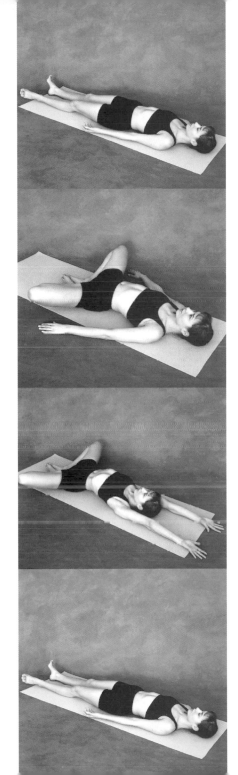

THE CORE PRACTICE

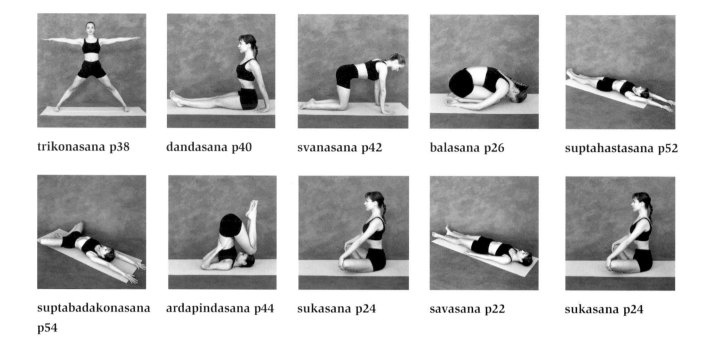

trikonasana p38   dandasana p40   svanasana p42   balasana p26   suptahastasana p52

suptabadakonasana p54   ardapindasana p44   sukasana p24   savasana p22   sukasana p24

This practice can be used for relaxation and rejuvenation.

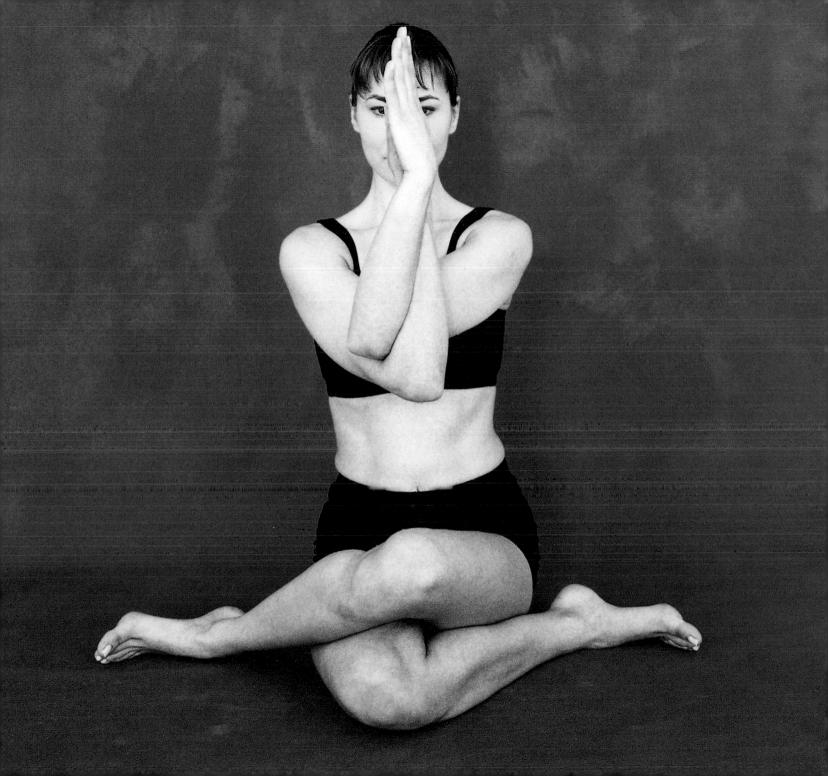

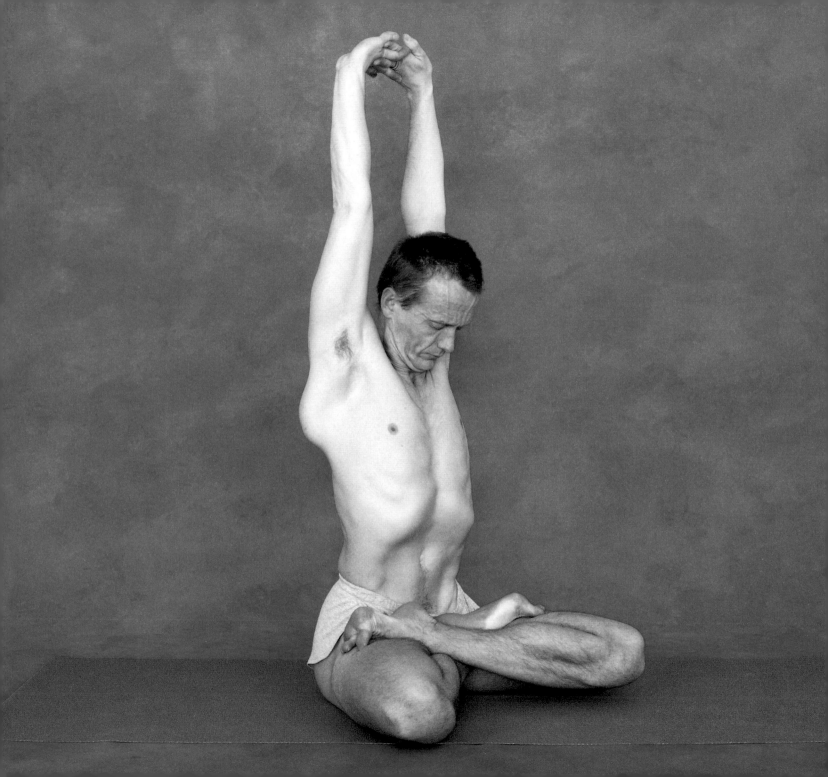

THE BANDHAS

The bandhas provide the integrating structural and energetic dynamic of yoga practice. Without them yoga postures are mere posturing. They may promote flexibility, strength, structural enhancement even, but they will not be spiritual practice. A spiritual practice is any process that brings you to the actuality of your true nature. The means may be varied, but the process is always the same. To arrive at your authentic, unconditioned nature you must first journey and see through your imagined, supposed, conditioned nature. Spiritual practice is symbolized by the image of the lotus blossom. Its beauty flowers out of the grime of the mud. So it is for us. If we are to access and express our true nature, rather than just act out an imitation of it based on hearsay and guesswork, we have to go down into the dross that has covered it up.

The bandhas are the means whereby we initiate this process in hatha yoga. They internalize our energy, our awareness and the effect of our practice; they unify the body structurally and energetically; they unify the body and mind; and they clarify, challenge, develop and eventually release the breath. But most important of all, the bandhas generate the momentum and energy that allows us to confront and burn up our imposed limitations. They do this by containing, transforming and redirecting our energy and attention. They contain the energy generated through the postures in the trunk, by sealing it at the top and bottom. They intensify and transform this energy by circulating it powerfully within this container. They then redirect it into our core.

There are three aspects to this process: jalandharabandha (net supporting regulator or throat lock), uddiyanabandha (upwards flying regulator or abdominal lock) and mulabandha (root regulator or root lock). However, these three switches or locks work together as one. They are always unified in their application during the practice of the yoga postures with a few notable exceptions. When using the word lock to describe the bandhas it is important to understand the word lock as something that you open, rather than something that you close. Otherwise you may get into the undermining habit of tightening the muscles in the pelvic floor, abdomen and throat and thereby completely prevent the possibility of the bandhas. They are not aggressive manipulations of gross external muscles. They are subtle switching of energy regulators. The switching is done by muscular activity, of course, but not in an aggressive, closing way. It is done in a subtle, opening way. Through the application of the bandhas you are opening your spiritual doorway – activating the conduit to the divine that the softness of your core opens up.

When we are being challenged by a posture, from stiffness, weakness or tiredness, it is only too easy to lose the subtle attentiveness required of the bandhas. These subtle muscular grips then become coarse and aggressive and, instead of dynamizing the softness of the core, they tighten it, close it down and create tension all the way up the axis from the anus into the brain. Nothing can be more undermining of yoga practice than this deeply held state of tension. To prevent it, continuous awareness of the soft, passive quality of our core is absolutely necessary. It is onto this backdrop that we apply the bandhas.

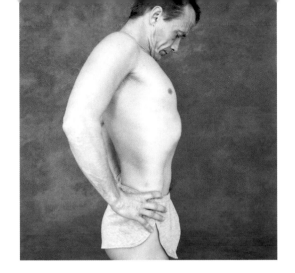

Jalandharabandha is an adjustment of the throat. Light contact is made between the top palate and the back of the throat. This contact does not create a complete blockage of the throat, as air can still pass to the sides. But it does interfere with the flow of air, slowing it down and making it more audible. The sound of the air passing should be smooth and soft, not rough and harsh. The breath should not be pulled in or pushed out. The respiratory muscles should be allowed to activate and release freely without any imposed conditions other than the bandhas. This contact replicates the state of the throat when the chin is down on the breastbone, as in shoulderstand variations. This is full jalandharabandha (shown above). In yoga postures where the chin is not on the chest, we apply internal jalandharabandha by adjusting the throat into this shape from the muscles in the throat itself. It is a little as if you were about to enunciate the word 'go', but stopped just before releasing air forward against the contact the palate has made with the throat for the 'g' sound to be possible. This is then held throughout the practice. After a while it will happen naturally as soon as you begin to practice. Jalandharabandha immediately induces an internalization of awareness and energy that can instantly be felt. After practising in this way it becomes impossible not to, as the comparative feeling of superficial externality is so obviously inappropriate to the purpose of hatha yoga.

Jalandharabandha is the easiest of the three bandhas. This does not mean that it is unimportant. Its external function is to slow the breathing down and make it audible. The sound of the breath acts like a mantra, soothing and detaching the mind from its preoccupation with external stimuli. Jalandharabandha, then, is a necessary aspect of the internalization of awareness that distinguishes yoga from other activities. The subtle function of jalandharabandha is to contain the energy generated by yoga postures and uddiyanabandha within the trunk. If this energy is allowed to pass upwards, the mind can become overstimulated and intensify its patterns of conditioned neurosis.

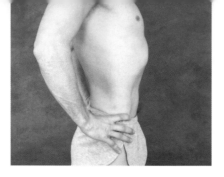

Uddiyanabandha is an adjustment *on* the abdomen. The abdominal wall and organs are drawn in and up, towards the spine and lungs. This makes the abdomen long, hollow and empty. Because it is lengthening, the external muscles of the abdomen become more firm. This is a passive response to the lengthening, however. It is not the result of contraction of these muscles. They *must* remain passive for uddiyanabandha to occur. The abdominal muscles and organs are being acted upon from above. They themselves are passive, although their position, shape and quality is completely transformed. The muscles that are being activated are in the chest. These are the very muscles that we would use to make a deep and full inhalation. They are applied continuously, however, regardless of whether we are breathing in or out. This makes the exhalation used during yoga practice feel a little like an inhalation, in that the chest is kept high and broad by the activation of these muscles of uddiyanabandha. To feel this, empty the lungs normally. Then, without allowing any air into the lungs, activate the chest as if you were taking in as much air as you possibly could. When the inhalation muscles are strong enough and used to this action, you will feel a hollowing at the solar plexus as it is sucked gently in. When the chest has reached its maximum height and breadth, allow the air to come in. This 'grip' you have created will create resistance to the inhalation as the lift of the solar plexus resists the downwards movement of the diaphragm. This resistance slows the inhalation down. When you start to breathe out, maintain this grip on the chest as strongly as you can throughout the exhalation. This will create a strong resistance to the exhalation, which naturally slows it down. It is in this way that the breath is slowed down in yoga breathing – from the bandhas, not from direct manipulation of the firing rate and rhythm of the respiratory muscles. The muscles that you are using to engage uddiyanabandha are behind and above the abdomen. This process is, in fact, a partial uddiyanabandha, as full uddiyanabandha requires empty lungs.

Full uddiyanabandha is traditionally done as a stand-alone practice, before sun salutations at the beginning of practice. It is a mock inhalation activated after fully emptying the lungs. Air is not allowed into the lungs and, as the

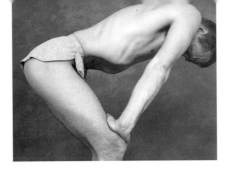

space inside the chest expands and increases, the pressure drops strongly. This would normally cause air to be sucked into the chest. As this is being prevented, the abdominal organs are sucked towards the chest instead. This is why the abdomen must be kept passive, not tense or contracting – if it is, it will not lift. This is when people push or press the muscles back in imitation of uddiyanabandha. Such pressurized states in the abdominal, thoracic and cranial cavities are all wrong. There should be negative pressure in all three. Correct uddiyanabandha drops the cranial pressure, which is felt as a softening of the brain. To clarify what this means, make a strong complete exhalation, tightening the lower abdomen to fully empty the lungs. At the end of this process you will have and feel strong positive pressure in all three cavities – cranial, thoracic and abdominal. It is not a feeling you will want to maintain. When uddiyana-bandha is incorrectly done, positive pressure is created in the abdomen; this also affects the cranium, bringing tension to the brain and the cranial bones.

Uddiyana is the key bandha. When mature, it spontaneously triggers the other two. Its structural impact is to lengthen the trunk, spine, core and lower back. This helps release the breath. It also helps to prevent swayback and compression of the lumbar vertebrae. Its internal, energetic function is to generate thermal and subtle energy. This energy is then directed by mulabandha into the core to purify and open it. When this energy is not being fully inter-nalized by correct mulabandha it creates excessive amounts of heat and sweating.

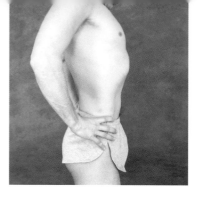

Mulabandha

Mulabandha is an adjustment *on* the pelvic floor. Like uddiyanabandha it is activated from above. The muscles of the pubic abdomen act on the pelvic floor, while the pelvic floor itself remains internally passive. The action of the muscles above, however, changes its position, shape and quality. This change can be misinterpreted as activity *in* the pelvic floor when, in fact, it is activity *on* the pelvic floor. The muscular action of mulabandha occurs by the groins, in the sloping lateral hollows running up from the edges of the pubic bone towards the hipbones. This area between the pubis and the hipbones is both abdominal and pelvic. It can be pushed forwards to clarify its edges. It is here that mulabandha occurs – within the area of the pelvic bones, although it also involves muscles extending into the abdomen. The muscular action of mulabandha is subtle, and is the only deliberate activation of abdominal muscles used in yoga postures. Any other activation of abdominal muscular activity will interfere with yoga breathing and prevent the internalization intended by the bandhas. Mulabandha is done by gently contracting the muscles by the groins, while keeping the rest of the pubic abdomen and central and upper abdomen completely passive. This occurs spontaneously with a deep and unforced exhalation. If you put your fingers in your groins you can feel a pencil-like line of muscle pushing gently but clearly up and out against your fingers, while the rest of the pubic abdomen between your fingers draws gently back without tightening. The anus should stay soft, although it will be lifted up and into the pelvic cavity which will make it narrower. DO NOT TIGHTEN YOUR ANUS if you can help it, if you can't help it, be aware of that and keep trying. (Awareness of failure is often the first step towards success.) The line of muscle that should be gently pushing up against your fingertips is angled outwards as it goes up, following the line of the groins.

This is the external action of mulabandha. It should broaden the back of the pelvis and engage the sacrum, keeping it stable and safe during your practice. It should also lift the pelvic floor into the pelvis and draw the mouth of the cervix in. While both the perineum itself and the cervical mouth can be drawn in without engaging the pubic abdomen, this is not enough to ensure the structural impact of mulabandha necessary to the safety of the spine. The effect of mulabandha on the sacrum should not be confused with the tucking action of the pelvic tilt, which is used to keep the lower back long in some exercise programmes. This does not engage or protect the sacrum. Moreover, it creates an energetic barrier between the legs and back, so that whatever is being done by the feet and legs is not transmitted to the spine, where it is required. Mulabandha also stabilizes the lungs and diaphragm, allowing the lungs to open more fully on activation of the respiratory muscles of inhalation. More important still is its energetic impact, which is to redirect the energy generated by the yoga postures and uddiyanabandha inwardly to purify and open the core. This can be felt as an instantaneous release of pressure and presence in the brain. When mulabandha is mature it feels as if the physical body is no longer a limitation, but opens up into its internal infinite dimensionlessness.

The integrated dynamic of the three bandhas is spirallic in its kinetic momentum. This spirallic charge can be felt as a strong internal upwards movement in the core and a more subtle downwards movement on the skin of the trunk. This spirallic charge must then be resonated throughout the whole body. It is taken out into the hands and feet through the limbs. The hands and feet then act as seals, sending the energy of uddiyanabandha back to the perineum and into the core. If the whole body is not engaged as an expression of the bandhas, then energy is dissipated and the mind tends to fragment and wander.

The hands replicate the bandhas by broadening across the base of the fingers and lengthening along the fingers. The palm then becomes hollow like the abdomen and the bases of the fingers become broad like the chest.

The feet replicate the bandhas by broadening across the ball of the foot and lengthening through the inner and front ankle and the Achilles tendon. The instep then becomes hollow like the abdomen, while the ball of the foot becomes broad and full like the chest.

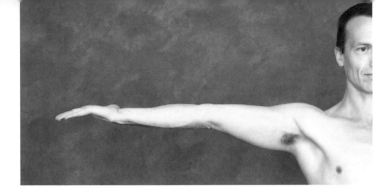

The spirallic dynamic of the bandhas is expressed in the arms by opposing the direction of movement of the ball of the thumb (downwards as the arm lengthens) to the direction of movement of the biceps (upwards as the arm lengthens). Combined with the activation of the hands – which sucks the muscles of the forearm in – this makes the arms long, by opening the joints, and strong, by twisting them to give them the tensile strength of a rope.

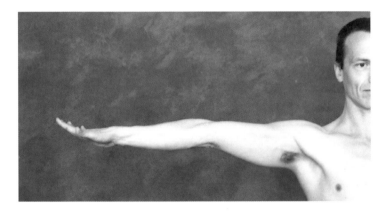

The spirallic dynamic of the bandhas is expressed in the legs by opposing the backwards movement of the inner ankle to the backwards movement of the outer hip. Combined with the sucking in of the thigh muscles and the activation of the feet, this makes the legs long, by opening the joints, and strong, by stabilizing them with a twisting motion that gives them the tensile strength of a rope.

It is important to develop the bandhas together. If jalandhara is absent or weak, the energy generated by uddiyana can overstimulate the brain and mind. If mula is absent or weak, uddiyana can dissipate energy in heat and dripping sweat. If uddiyana is absent or weak, it is not yoga.

ardasarvangasana

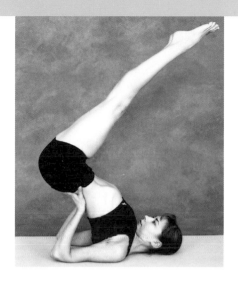

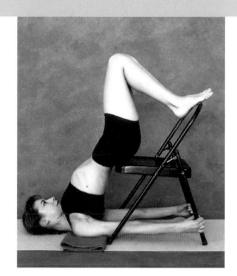

The half-shoulderstand is a brilliant posture in which to clarify the dynamic of the bandhas. As an inversion it is restful and refreshing. Its shape naturally facilitates and enhances the bandhas. The position of the head relative to the chest facilitates and enhances thoracic breathing and engages jalandharabandha. When in it, the focus should be on learning how to breathe freely and fully from the bandhas. This means watching the relationship between the abdominal wall and the ribcrests. Rather than the ribcrest remaining static while the abdomen puffs out and sinks back in, the ribcrests should flare out as you inhale and narrow again as you exhale. At the same time, the abdomen will rise as the ribs flare, although it should not puff up above the line of the ribs. Towards the end of the inhalation, effort must be made to keep the breath coming into the top lungs and prevent the abdomen from puffing. This is a definite challenge to the residual inertia of the top lungs, and it stimulates and develops their natural function.

Half-shoulderstand teaches how to use the arms and shoulders as the foundation of an inversion. It rests and rejuvenates the body, develops the wrists and arms, stimulates thoracic breathing and gives the spine an easy and gentle backbend. Make sure there is no pressure on any of the vertebrae and do not strain the neck muscles by lifting too hard and high. In addition, ensure that your back is not rounding as it would in embryo pose. If it is, lift your top spine and chest towards you, while rolling your pelvis away from your face, bringing more weight onto your hands.

In the beginning it is likely that your hands, wrists or arms will become tired as a result of the support they are giving to the pelvis and legs. It then becomes necessary to alternate between the half-shoulderstand and the embryo pose to rest them. Alternatively, you can dedicate a whole session to exploring the bandhas in half-shoulderstand on a chair.

The half-shoulderstand is a key posture in the process of learning yoga. It has many important functions besides being a perfect place to clarify the dynamic of the bandhas. First, as an inversion it rests the cellular structure of the whole body from the pull of gravity. This is deeply rejuvenating for the whole body and at the root of the immense restorative benefits to be gained from inversions. It also teaches the correct lift of the back, necessary to a safe full shoulderstand and its variations. This is achieved by the correct use of the arms and hands in lifting the vertebrae of the spine and neck just off the floor so there is no pressure on them. This requires a definite and continuous dynamic in the arms and shoulders, which are pressed down as the foundation of the posture. If the full shoulderstand and its variations are practised without this lift they can irritate and even injure the neck and spine.

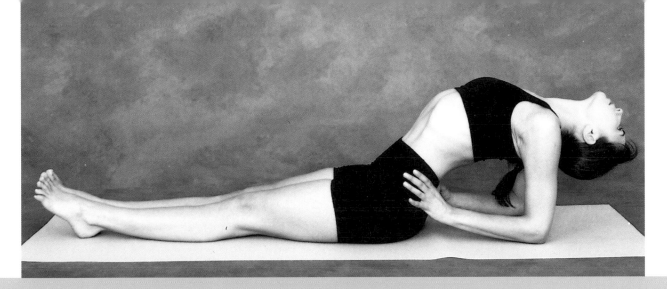

ardamatsyasana

Half-fish is the counterpose to the effect of the half-shoulderstand on the neck. It also takes the spine into the same gentle backbend as the half-shoulderstand. It relieves the neck from any pressure or strain that may inadvertently have been put on the neck and spine by not activating the correct lift in half-shoulderstand. It also helps to clarify the bandhas and stimulate the correct method of inhalation.

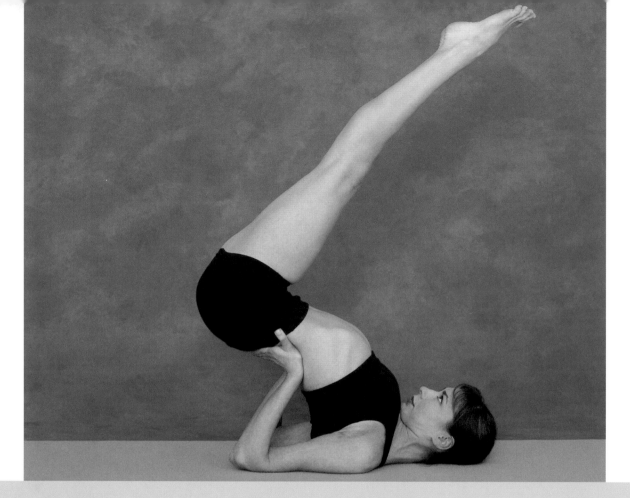

ardasarvangasana

This posture is the key inversion. The position of the head naturally stimulates jalandharabandha. Maintain a strong foundation with the shoulders, upper arm and elbows. Use this to keep the spinal vertebrae off the floor. Keep the neck long, shoulders away from the ears. Most people need to keep the hands under the pelvis and not under the back, or it will be hard to give the spine and abdomen the correct line and quality. Focus on the bandhas with your abdomen passive, long and hollow; solar plexus sucked in; chest broad and active; pubic abdomen flat and broad; anus soft.

- Lie on your back, arms and legs outstretched, shoulders away from your ears.
- **Bend your legs and draw your feet close to your buttocks, knees together.**
- Extend your arms past your buttocks. Press your palms firmly into the floor.
- **Pushing with your hands, roll your knees up towards your chest so your buttocks and lower back rise away from the floor.**
- Bring your hands up to support your back while lowering your knees to your forehead. Soften your core, allowing anus, eyes, ears, tongue and brain to be completely passive.
- **Slip your hands underneath the pelvic rim as you roll your pelvis away from your face so the knees lift away from your head, bringing all the weight of your legs and pelvis onto your hands.**
- Roll your pubic bone and hipbones as far away from your face as you can, making your abdomen as long as possible.
- **Press down with your elbows and forearms and, broadening your shoulders, gently lift the vertebrae just off the floor so there is no pressure on them.**
- Arch your back so that the top spine moves into your body and the chest opens and lifts towards your face, bringing the breastbone into more direct contact with your chin. Do not press the chin forwards.
- **Broaden and flatten your pubic abdomen and engage mulabandha, keeping your anus soft. Straightening your legs, suck your thigh muscles into the bones, and broaden the heels and balls of your feet while lengthening their inner and outer edges.**
- Flatten and lengthen your abdomen, sucking your solar plexus in so that the ribcrests activate and broaden. Keep the abdominal muscles passive by engaging uddiyanabandha.

Hold the posture – with your abdomen passive, long and hollow; solar plexus sucked in; chest broad and active; pubic abdomen, flat and broad. Allow the anus, eyes, ears, tongue and brain to be completely passive. Watch the dynamic movement of your ribcrests and keep the abdominal wall from puffing out. When ready to release, do so by reversing the steps you used to enter (without necessarily synchronizing with your breath).

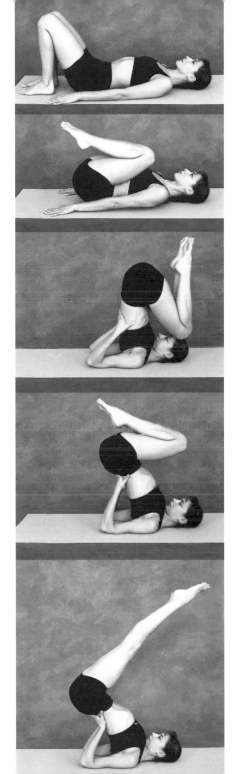

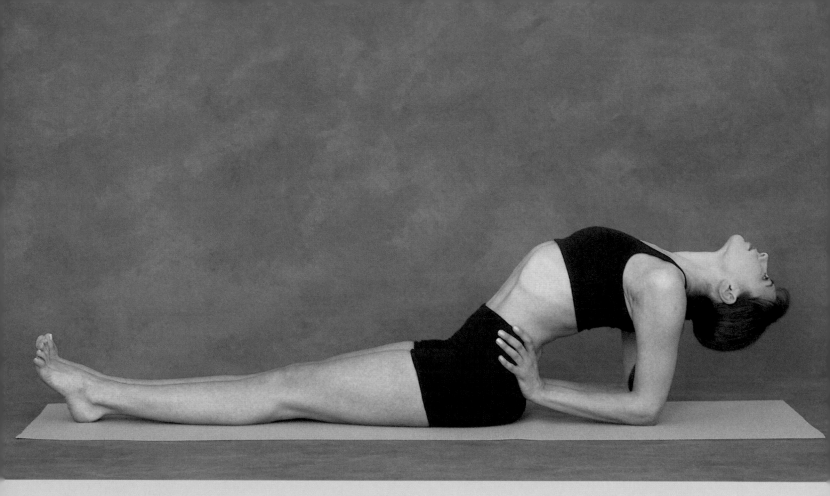

ardamatsyasana

This posture releases the neck and is the counterpose to the half-shoulderstand. If you find you are unable to release your neck, and it is uncomfortable, take the chin back to the chest. Keep the legs and feet dynamic and grounding you. Keep the lower back soft. When you take the head up and back, roll the shoulders forwards to lengthen and release the neck. Get a good lift into this action from the base of the skull. Focus on the bandhas with your abdomen passive, long and hollow; solar plexus sucked in; chest broad and active; pubic abdomen flat and broad; anus soft.

- Sit with your legs relaxed in front of you.
- **Align the hips and bring your inner heels together with legs still relaxed.**
- Bring the balls of the big toes and the inner anklebones in contact with each other, so that the inner and outer edges of the feet are the same distance away from you.
- **Suck the thigh muscles into the thighbones so that the kneecaps are pulled up and in, the knee bones go down and the shin and thigh bones line up.**
- Broaden the balls of your feet, allowing the centre of each to lead away from your ankle and not the ball of the big toe.
- **Lengthen the front ankle, Achilles tendon and inner ankle.**
- Soften your core, allowing anus, eyes, ears, tongue and brain to be completely passive. Lean back onto your elbows, placing your hands on your hips, thumbs to the back, fingers the front.
- **Keeping your legs engaged and pressing down, broaden and flatten your pubic abdomen and engage mulabandha, keeping your anus soft.**
- Pressing down with your elbows, flatten and lengthen your abdomen, suck your solar plexus in so that the ribcrests activate and broaden, engaging uddiyana-bandha. Keeping your abdominal muscles passive, lift your top spine into your chest, so your chest opens, broadens and lifts.
- **Moving from the base of your skull, gently rotate your chin forward and up, keeping the back of your neck soft and free.**
- **Take your chin back in an arc as you allow your head to drop gently towards your back.**

Hold the posture – abdomen passive, long and hollow; solar plexus sucked in; chest broad and active; pubic abdomen flat and broad. Allow the anus, eyes, ears, tongue and brain to be completely passive. Keep your feet alive, legs active, while aware of the free flow of inhalation and exhalation. Release when you feel ready to.

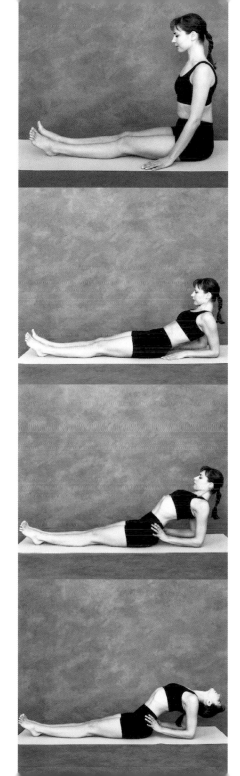

THE BANDHA PRACTICE

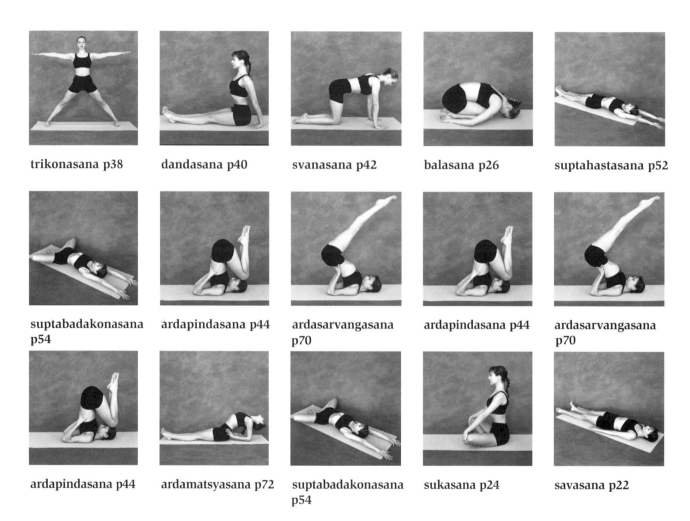

trikonasana p38

dandasana p40

svanasana p42

balasana p26

suptahastasana p52

suptabadakonasana p54

ardapindasana p44

ardasarvangasana p70

ardapindasana p44

ardasarvangasana p70

ardapindasana p44

ardamatsyasana p72

suptabadakonasana p54

sukasana p24

savasana p22

This practice can be used for relaxation and rejuvenation.

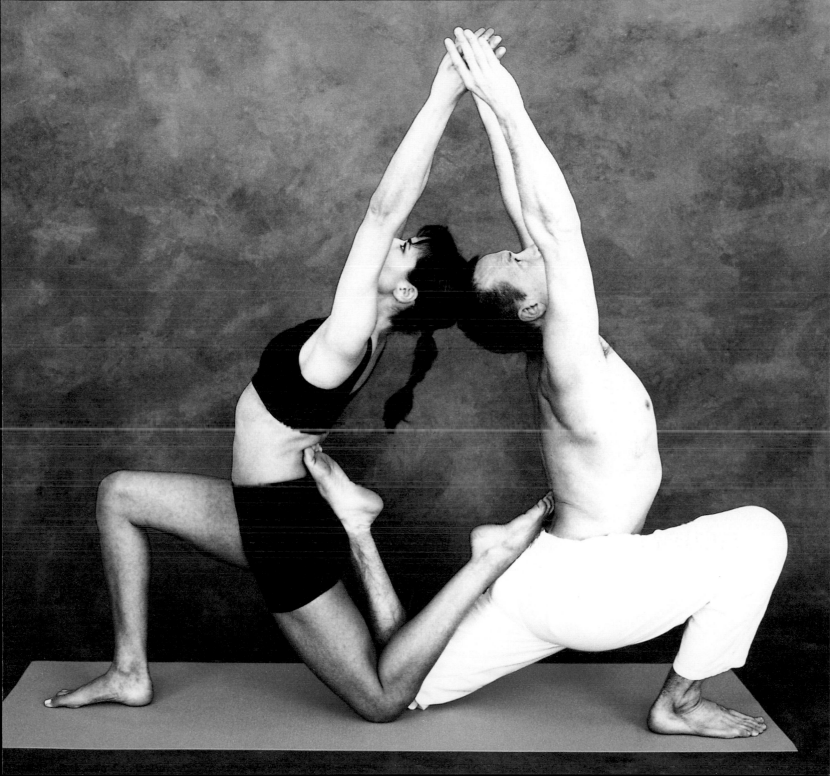

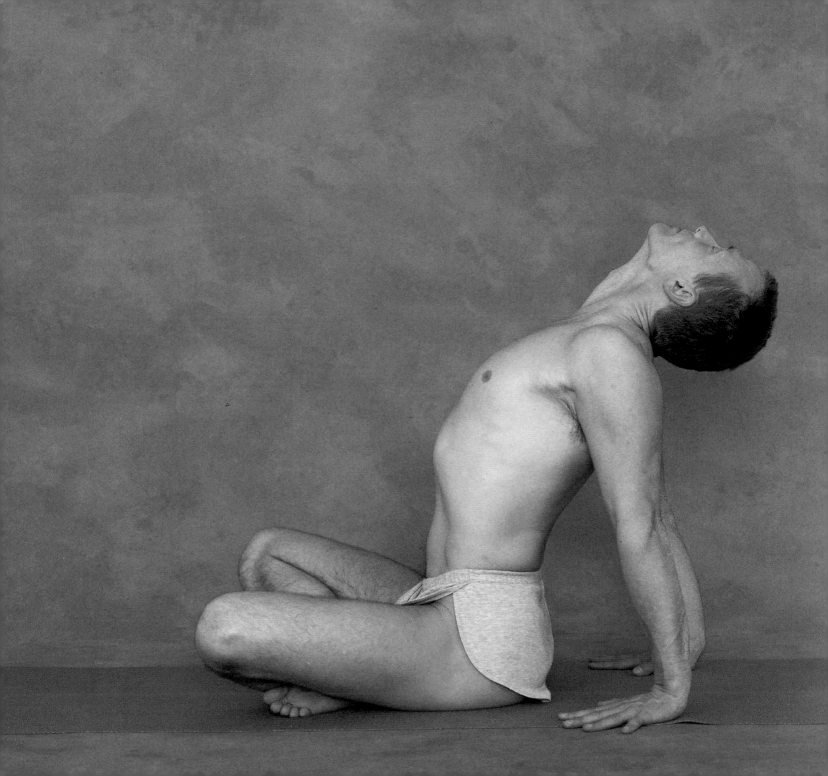

ENGAGING THE ARMS AND HANDS

The arms are active in almost all yoga postures. No matter what shape they take, whether they are straight, bent, wrapped around; no matter whether they function as supports or grips or extensions, they are always used to express the dynamic of the bandhas. By doing so they contribute to the energetic and structural integrity of the postures. They express the bandha dynamic by being activated spirically. This means that the biceps roll out away from the chest, while the forearm resists this motion by turning in the opposite direction. By opposing the momentum of the top and bottom of the arm to each other a strong charge is created in the arms. This charge is a direct expression of the charge that the bandhas generate in the trunk. It also has a similar function. It stabilizes the arms, making them stronger and more effective. It also energizes the arms, making them more alive, responsive and communicative. This allows them to transmit the energetic quality and effects of the bandhas to the hands. It also creates space in the wrist, elbow and shoulder joints so that the arms lengthen and lighten. At the same time, circulation of blood, lymph and vitality improves. In hatha yoga the arms can be seen and used as extensions of the lungs. Correct use of the arms opens the chest, engages the top spine and stimulates more free and full breathing.

The hands also always express the dynamic of the bandhas – no matter whether they are bearing weight, holding on or free. They do this by lengthening through the fingers and broadening across the finger bases. The fingers are allowed to be slightly apart without pulling them away from each other. It is easy to overwork the hands and fingers, creating tension. When they are activated correctly they will feel alive, responsive and communicative. They are then able to express the energetic quality of the bandhas and participate in the structural and energetic integrity of the postures. They also mirror the function and effect of the bandhas by acting as seals at the extremities, containing energy and redirecting it back to the core, via mulabandha. The action of the hands draws and returns energy at the same time. This can be clearly felt.

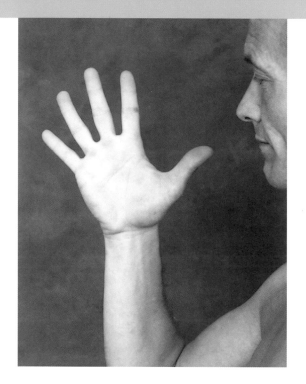

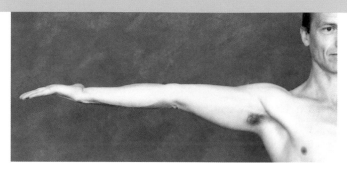

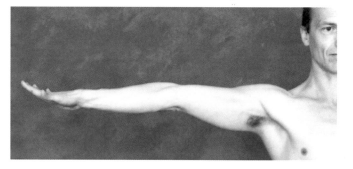

It is only a convenient linguistic and conceptual convention to separate hand from arm. In actuality, in our actual experience of them, it is not possible to draw up a clear or consistent boundary between them. They are functionally and experientially indivisible. This can be clearly felt if you pay attention to the quality, shape and dimensions of the muscles of the forearm as you lengthen your fingers and broaden your palms. The muscle of your forearm will engage and suck into the bone. This is the same effect that you are looking for when you suck the thigh muscles in. Likewise, the arms cannot in actuality be separated from the trunk. By engaging the arms spiralically the deltoids and chest broaden, the lungs open and the breath flows more freely. The activity of the arms then is nothing other than a direct, extended continuation of the activity of the bandhas in process and in effect.

To understand the spirallic dynamic of the arms you have only to stretch one out from your shoulder, parallel to the floor. In doing so, make your arms straight and as long as you can. Lengthen the fingers and broaden the palms, feeling the forearms engage. Then, being aware of changes in the chest and deltoid, roll the palm slowly upwards and establish more length in the arm. As you do this, feel the sensations of the biceps gripping into the bone and the sensation of opening and lightening in the elbow and shoulder. You can also feel the chest broadening and opening.

Maintaining the dynamic in the chest, shoulder joint, biceps and elbow, and keeping the fingers long and the palm broad, revolve the wrist back over without changing the line of the upper arm at all. This requires concentration but is not difficult to do. You will then feel the forearm coming alive in a similar way to the upper arm. The muscles will grip into the bone and you will feel a contrasting openness in the wrist.

The arm is now spiralling – expressing the dynamic of the bandhas. The muscular grip on the bone and the opening of the joint both stimulate circulation. The twisting form of the arm gives it strength and stability as whole, while giving it openness and ease in the joints. This enables stability to be established without sacrificing comfort. This dynamic should not produce any tension or hardness in the arm, face or brain. Make sure you are not aggressive with the fingers or the rotating movements of the arm. This spirallic action is established whenever the arms are active.

adomukasvanasana

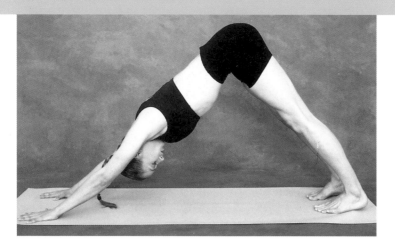

Downwards-dog pose teaches the spirallic activity of the arms, and especially how this opens the chest. When the upper arms are rotated away from the shoulders the top spine is taken in and the chest broadens. You may hear a 'pop' or 'crack' as this happens. Don't worry, you have just become your own chiropractor. This will only happen if the armpits and chest do not collapse towards the floor. A strong, external, upwards dynamic must be maintained in the upper arm so that this not only turns the biceps but also keeps the chest lifting away from the floor. A common problem in this posture is to push the head down to the floor and collapse the chest and armpits. This closes the lungs, strains the shoulders and destroys the structural and energetic integrity of the posture. Although the focus in this lesson is on the arms, the legs must be worked also.

Downwards-dog also teaches the internal dynamic of postural integrity. It awakens the intelligence of the body evenly across all the planes. It allows the dualities of the body to be easily harmonized and transcended. It clarifies the use of the limbs in supporting and activating the trunk. It is a restful, refreshing posture once you can establish it in comfortable stability. It develops the arms, legs, hands and feet. It releases the pelvis and the spine, as well as softening the back. It also rests the heart, rejuvenates the legs, opens the chest and aligns the top spine. It is a key posture in the practice of hatha yoga. It can be used to awaken the whole body as a gentle warm up. It can also be used as a dynamic resting place, but only when it can be done without strain or stress.

trikonasana

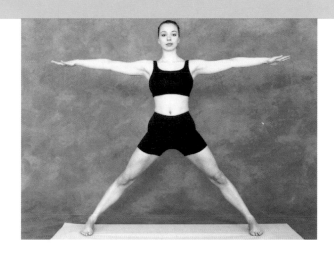

Triangle pose is a brilliant posture for clarifying the spirallic action of the arms. The arms must lengthen out of the armpits, with the palms broadening and the fingers lengthening. The upper arm rolls up and back, and the wrist is held down by an opposing rotation through the pad of the thumb. Detailed instructions for this posture are given on page 39.

dandasana

Staff pose also requires the spirallic action of the arms, with the hands pressing firmly down. The spiral is initiated from the downward pressure of the base of the index finger. Detailed instructions for this posture are given on page 41.

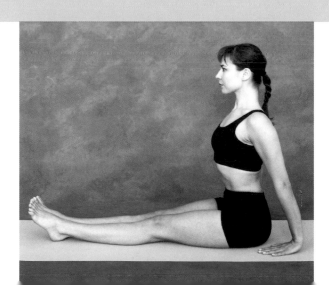

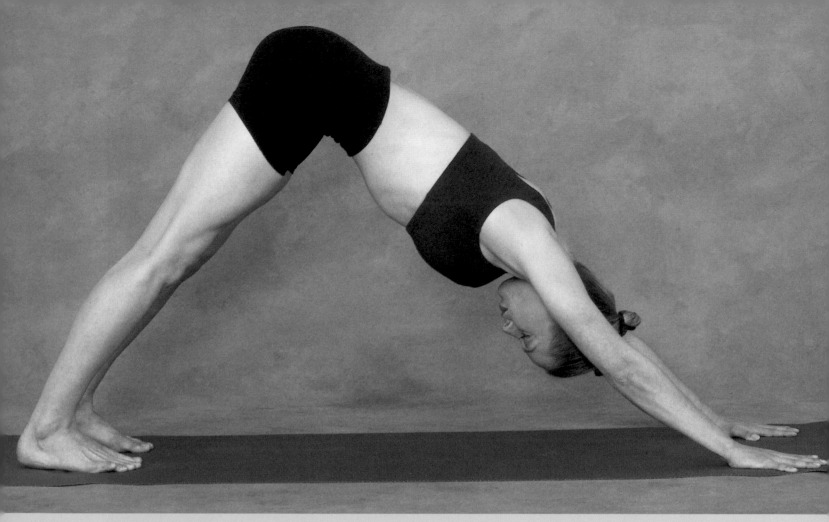

adomukasvanasana

Keep the action, and your awareness, even: hands and feet, arms and legs, left and right, top and bottom, front and back. Use the bandhas to lengthen the trunk, spine and core. Even if the heels do not make it to the floor, do not walk the feet in. This will distort the integrity and effect of the posture by rounding the back, inhibiting the bandhas and shortening the spine and core. Yoga is not about taking the line of least resistance to make a poor imitation of a geometric shape. Ground the bases of the index fingers and turn the biceps out, taking the shoulders away from your ears.

- **Settle comfortably into balasana and soften your core.**
- Elongate your arms out of your shoulders in front of you, with the hands shoulder-width apart.
- **Press your hands firmly down into the floor, lengthening the fingers and broadening across the base of the fingers.**
- Keeping the bases of the index fingers grounded, roll the biceps up and out, away from your ears so that the outer elbow bones roll down towards the floor, as the arms move away from the neck.
- **Pushing from the bases of the index fingers, lift your buttocks off your heels and straighten the legs, taking the hips into the air. Allow your head to drop down towards the floor and, with neck relaxed, look back between your feet.**
- Pivot your hipbones towards your thighs and flatten and lengthen your abdomen, sucking your solar plexus in so that the ribcrests activate and broaden. Keep your abdominal muscles passive.
- **Roll your pubic bone back, broaden and flatten your pubic abdomen and engage mulabandha, keeping your anus soft.**
- Make your feet alive by broadening the balls of the feet and the heel and lengthening the inner and outer edges. Take the heels down towards the floor.
- **Suck your thigh muscles into the bones and make the legs strong.**

Hold the posture with the bandhas engaged, feeling the free flow of your breath, keeping the trunk long, legs strong and a strong spirallic dynamic in the arms – until ready to release. Release back to balasana.

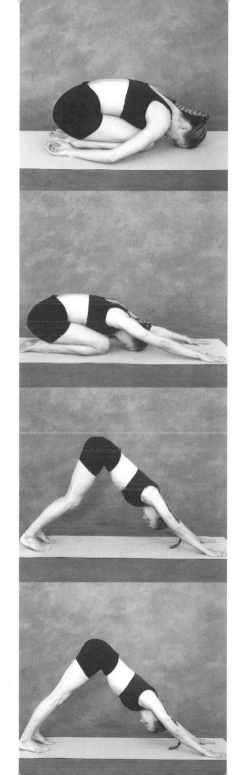

THE DOWNWARDS-DOG PRACTICE

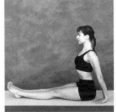

svanasana p42

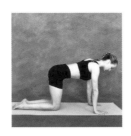

adomukasvanasana p82

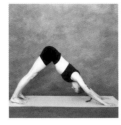

svanasana p42

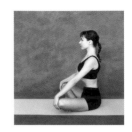

adomukasvanasana p82

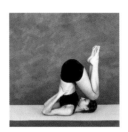

sukasana p24

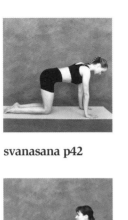

dandasana p40

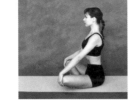

sukasana p24

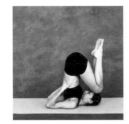

ardapindasana p44

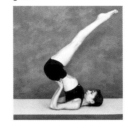

ardasarvangasana p70

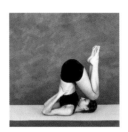

ardapindasana p44

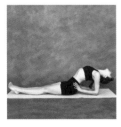

ardamatsyasana p72

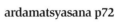

savasana p22

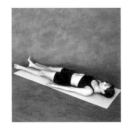

sukasana p24

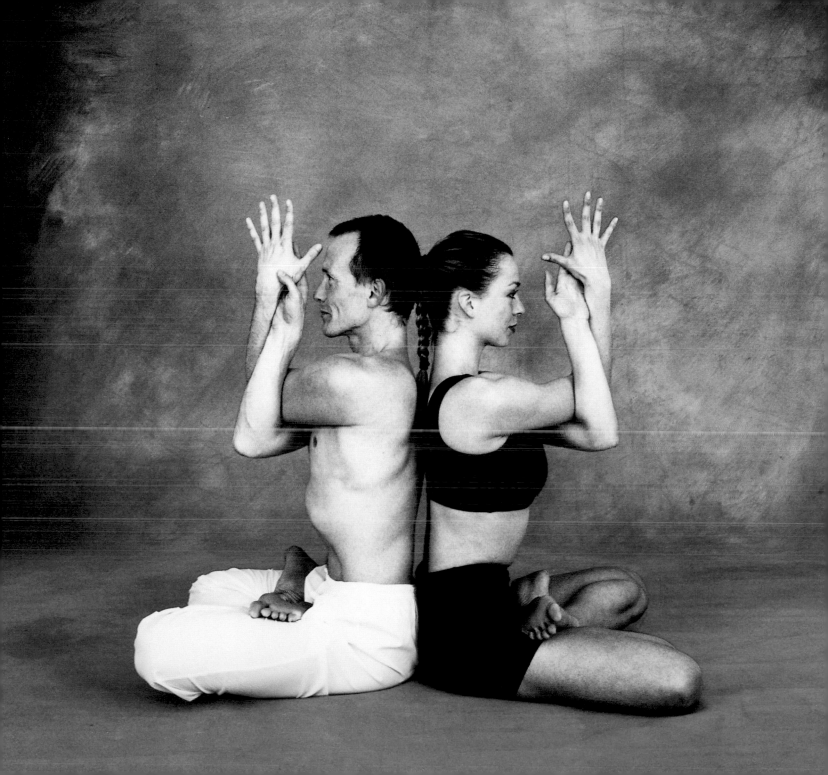

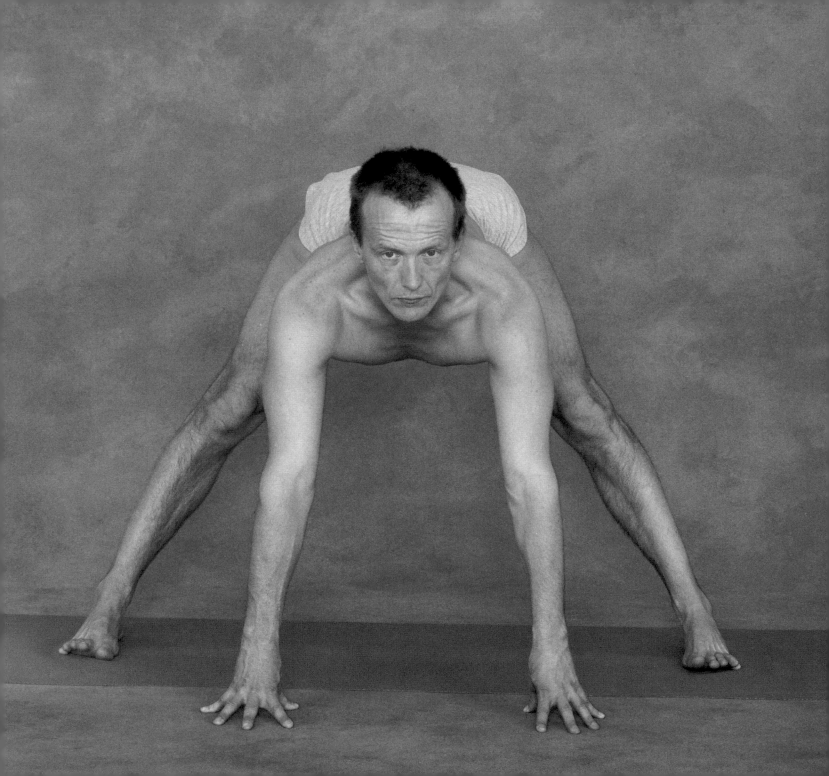

ENGAGING THE LEGS AND FEET

The inherent activity of both the legs and the feet in yoga postures is to express and support the dynamic of the bandhas. This means that both feet and the legs are activated spiralically. In the feet this means that the broadening and lengthening of the feet is part of a double helix. This double helix, or spirallic action of the feet is a constant. It is applied to the feet at all times, except in the rare instances when the feet are deliberately allowed to be completely passive. It is activated in the following, simple manner. Pressing down with the ball of the big toe, broaden the ball of the foot across to the ball of the little toe, then lengthen the outer edge of the foot back to the outer heel. This is the external spiral of the feet. Maintaining that dynamic, pressing down with the ball of the big toe, lengthen back along the inner edge of the feet to the inner heel and broaden out from there to the outer heel. This is the internal spiral of the feet. They are supposed to balance each other – to take the feet beyond the differentiations of dualities such as left/right, front/back etc. In practice, however, we have to vary the emphasis according to the structure and habits of our own feet and the posture we are in. Sometimes the posture and the habit of our feet favour the internal spiral. If this is the case, we have to give extra emphasis to the external spiral. Or vice versa. Some postures tend to show the same pattern amongst almost all students. Some show a greater variety. It is vital to remember then that generalized postural instructions may not apply to you (your teacher may not even realize this). So be careful that you are not working the wrong way for your structure. This happens more often that you might think. When you develop a sound sense of the spirallic dynamic of adjustment, and the intention of going beyond dualistic differentiations in your body awareness, then you can guide yourself effectively.

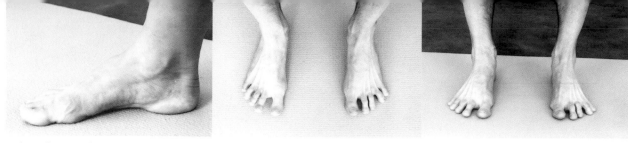

broadening the heels spiralically   **broadening the balls of the feet spiralically**   **feet spirals balanced**

This spirallic action in the feet carries up as a double helix into the legs. This is much harder to feel and adjust than the feet spirals. It depends on two things. First, that your legs can straighten, and second, that you can engage the leg muscles into the bone without making them bulge from aggressive contraction (this was focused on in Lesson Two). When this becomes more possible, the spirallic action of the legs will also. When the legs are free of tension and their intelligence awakened, they will respond automatically to the spiralling of the feet if they are engaged correctly. Nothing more need be done. Until then, however, we can work directly on the leg spirals themselves. This we do in a manner similar to that by which we spiral the arms. We oppose the top and the bottom of the leg to each other.

We feel this as a strong backward movement of the inner ankle bones and a balancing backwards movement of the outer knee. Again, both these actions are supposed to balance each other so that the leg becomes centred and stable within the hip socket. Either one can be overdone and distort the shape, position and functioning of the legs.

The external spiral of the feet and legs brings stability to the pelvis and thereby to the spine. The internal spiral of the feet and legs brings spaciousness to the pelvis and trunk. Together they nurture the stability and comfort that define yoga posture.

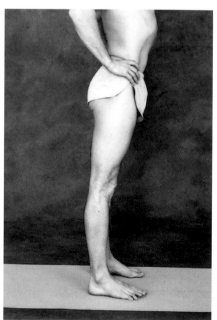

padottanasana

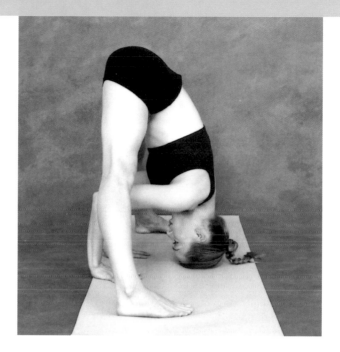

Leg-stretch pose is a continuation of trikonasana. It clarifies the spirallic dynamic of both feet and legs. It teaches the use of the feet and legs in moving the trunk into a forward extension. It also teaches how to create space between the legs to broaden the pelvic floor and stimulate mulabandha. As a forward extension of the spine, it challenges the bandhas, thereby refining them. The intermediate stage, urdvapadottanasana, or gazing pose, teaches how to clarify the bandhas and use them to support spinal extension. These two positions can be used dynamically, according to the principles outlined in the next lesson.

This posture develops the feet and legs and lengthens the hamstrings, while freeing the pelvis and releasing the back and spine. The external spirals of the feet (and legs) create grip in the outside of the pelvis, which supports the work of mulabandha and offers stability. The internal spirals of the feet create openness and softness in the groins and pelvic floor, and support the outwards action of the buttockbones that broaden the pelvic floor and supports uddiyanabandha. Mulabandha stabilizes and supports the sacrum, diaphragm and lungs. Uddiyanabandha stabilizes the lower back and abdomen, opens the chest and lengthens the spine and core.

uttanasana

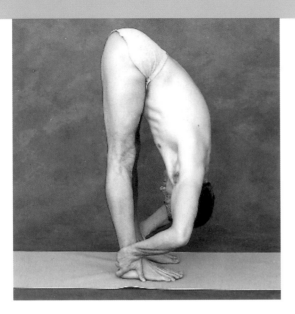

Standing fold is a more intense forward extension than padottanasana. It also teaches how to engage the legs and use the feet and legs to broaden the pelvic floor, and to support a forward extension. But being more intense, it is more challenging and therefore more potent than padottanasana. The intermediate stage, known as head-raised pose, teaches how to clarify the bandhas and use them to support spinal extension. These two positions can be used dynamically, according to the principles outlined in the next lesson. Standing fold clarifies the spirallic dynamic of both feet and legs. It also teaches how to create space between the legs to broaden the pelvic floor and stimulate mulabandha. As a forward extension of the spine, it challenges the bandhas, thereby refining them. Standing fold should never be released upwards with straight legs. Always release through its counterpose fierce pose, utktasana, as described in the instructions. Standing fold develops the feet and legs and lengthens the hamstrings, while freeing the pelvis and releasing the back and spine. The external spirals of the feet (and legs) create grip in the outside of the pelvis, and support the work of mulabandha by offering stability. The internal spirals of the feet create openness and softness in the groins and pelvic floor, and support uddiyanabandha. Mulabandha stabilizes and supports the sacrum, diaphragm and lungs. Uddiyanabandha stabilizes the lower back and abdomen, opens the chest and lengthens the spine and core.

adomukasvanasana

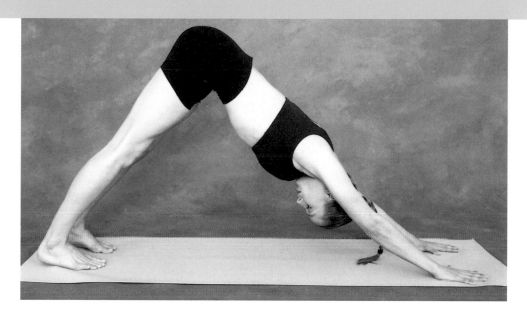

Downwards-dog pose is here used to teach the spirallic action of the legs. This is based on the spirallic activity of the feet, especially the broadening of the ball of the foot that this gives. For the legs to express the spirals of the feet they must be fully engaged, this means that the thigh and calf muscles must be sucking into the bone. The feet spirals can then be transmitted to the legs by moving the inner ankles and the outer knees backwards so that these two actions balance each other. Detailed instructions for this posture are given on page 83.

dandasana

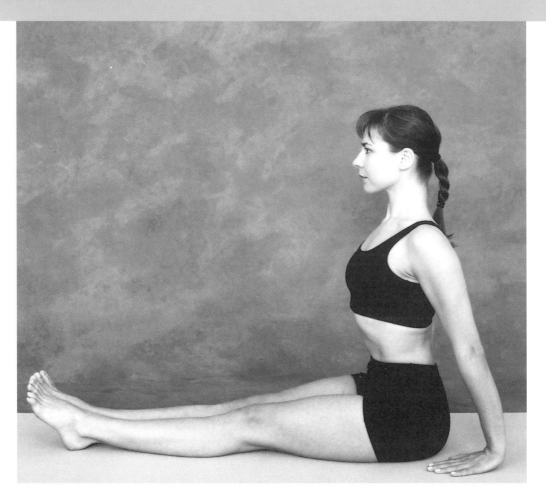

Staff pose   also requires the spirallic, grounding action of the legs. Press the heels down gently as you broaden the balls of your feet, while lengthening the front and inner ankles. Suck the thigh muscles into the bone and take the knees down. Detailed instructions for this posture are given on page 41.

ardasarvangasana

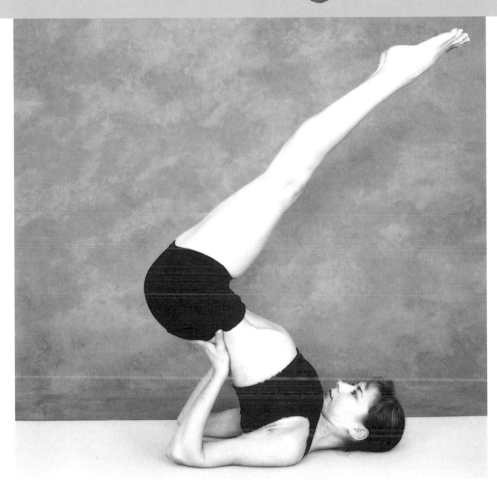

Half-shoulderstand also requires the spirallic action of the legs. Broaden the balls of your feet, while lengthening the front and inner ankles. Suck the thigh muscles into the bone and take the knees back. Detailed instructions for this posture are given on page 71.

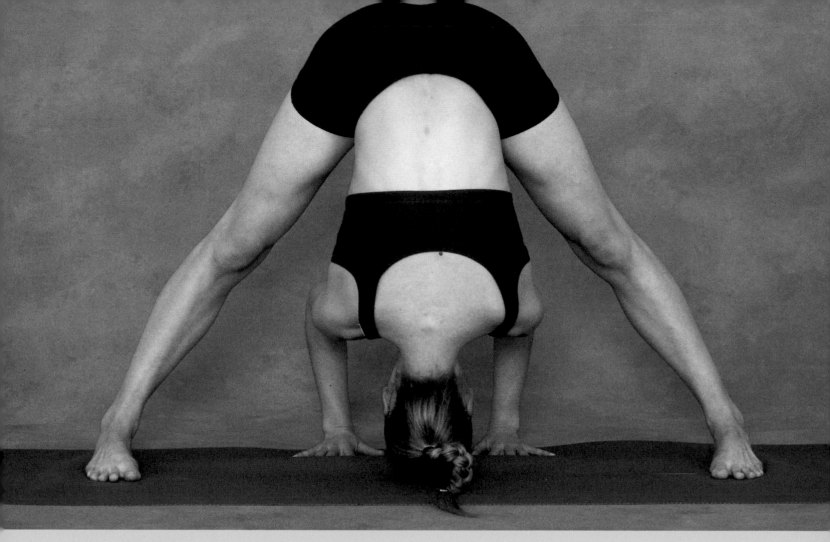

padottanasana

Keep the weight even between both feet, between the balls of the feet and the heels, and between the inner and outer edges of the feet. Keep the action even between the inner and outer spirals of feet and legs. Do not force the back down or in – the spine should be a continuous gentle curve. As well as being a surrendering of the spine, allow the forward extension to be an expression of the activity of the feet, legs, pelvic pivot, and the bandhas.

- Stand in trikonasana.
- **Suck the thigh muscles into your thighbones so that your legs become straight and strong but not tense. Ground the four corners of each foot – ball of the big toe, ball of the little toe, inner heel and outer heel – evenly and fully.**
- Internally spiral the feet, pressing back from the ball of the big toe to the inner heel and pressing from the inner heel to the outer heel in a rotating motion, keeping both feet firmly grounded.
- **Externally spiral the feet by pressing out from the ball of the big toe to the ball of the little toe, and lengthening the outer edge of the foot, pressing back from the ball of the little toe to the outer heel.**
- Internally spiral the legs by moving the inner ankle bones back so that the groins move backwards, softening them. Move the inner edges of the knees away from each other and broaden the pelvic floor.
- **Externally spiral the legs by moving the outer knees backwards, taking the outer hips back.**
- Engaging the bandhas, broaden and flatten your pubic abdomen, keeping the anus soft. Lengthen your abdomen, sucking your solar plexus in so that the ribcrests activate and broaden. Keep your abdominal muscles passive.
- **Pivoting your pelvis, with the legs and feet dynamically spiralling, take your fingertips to the floor underneath your shoulders.** If you cannot reach the floor, use a block, brick or book to place your hands on
- Spiralling your arms and legs, raise your head, and lengthen your arms, raising your armpits. Look ahead (urdvapadottanasana, gazing pose). Hold for as long as you wish and clarify the foot and leg spirals before going further.
- **Bend your arms and move your hands back so you can press them dynamically into the floor with arms spiralling. Relax your neck and drop the crown of your head towards the floor.**

Hold the posture – feet and legs spiralling, bandhas engaged, aware of the free flow of inhalation and exhalation – until ready to release.

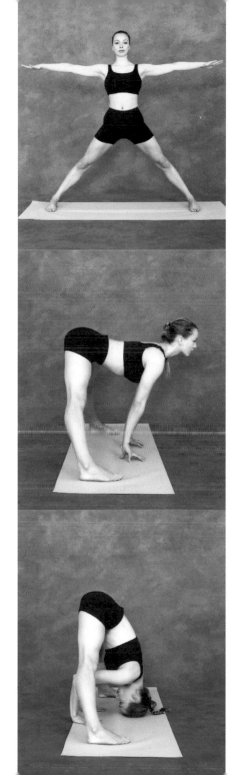

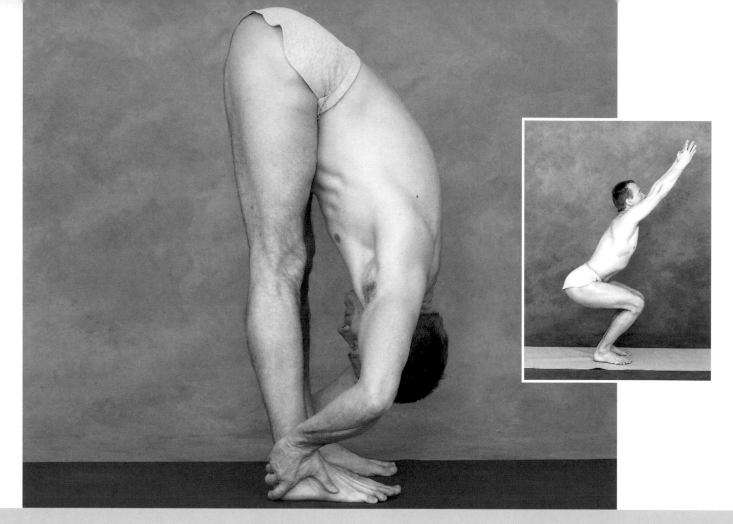

uttanasana

Keep the weight even between both feet, between the balls of the feet and the heels, and between the inner and outer edges of the feet. Keep the action even between the inner and outer spirals of feet and legs. Do not force the back down, in or straight – the spine should be a continuous gentle curve. As well as being a surrendering of the spine, allow the forward extension to be an expression of the activity of the feet, legs and pelvic pivot, and the bandhas. Remember to always release through utktasana or fierce pose (see inset picture).

- Stand with your feet parallel and slightly apart, hands on hips.
- **Suck the thigh muscles into your thighbones so that your legs become straight and strong but not tense. Ground the four corners of each foot – ball of the big toe, ball of the little toe, inner heel and outer heel – evenly and fully.**
- Internally spiral the feet, pressing back from the ball of the big toe to the inner heel and pressing from the inner heel to the outer heel in a rotating motion, keeping both feet firmly grounded.
- **Externally spiral the feet by pressing out from the ball of the big toe to the ball of the little toe, and lengthening the outer edge of the foot, pressing back from the ball of the little toe to the outer heel.**
- Internally spiral the legs by moving the inner ankle bones back so that the groins move backwards, softening them. Move the inner edges of the knees apart and broaden the pelvic floor.
- **Externally spiral the legs by moving the outer knees backwards, taking the outer hips back.**
- Engaging the bandhas, broaden and flatten your pubic abdomen, keeping your anus soft. Lengthen your abdomen, sucking your solar plexus in so that the ribcrests activate and broaden. Keep your abdominal muscles passive.
- **Pivoting your pelvis, with the legs and feet dynamically spiralling, take your hands to your ankles, fingers wrapping round the Achilles tendons to the inner ankles.**
- Spiralling your arms and legs, raise your head, and lengthen your arms, raising your armpits and look ahead. This is known as head-raised pose or arduttanasana.
- **Bending your arms, press your outer anklebones with the balls of your thumbs, wrapping your hands round the back ankles and pulling on the skin of the inner ankles with your fingers. Relax your neck and drop the crown of your head towards the floor as you lengthen your upper arms to lengthen the trunk. Keep the back and spine passive.**

Hold the posture – feet and legs spiralling, bandhas engaged, aware of the free flow of inhalation and exhalation – until ready to release. Release through the counterpose by bending your legs and raising your arms up in front of you as you inhale into fierce pose. Release fierce pose without holding on an exhalation back to standing upright.

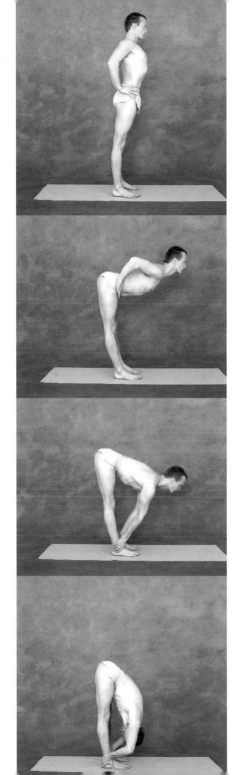

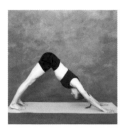

**adomukasvan-
asana p82**

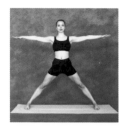

trikonasana p38

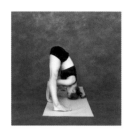

**urdvapadottan-
asana p95**

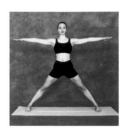

padottanasana p94

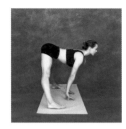

trikonasana p38

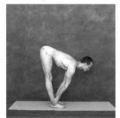

arduttanasana p97

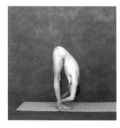

uttanasana p96

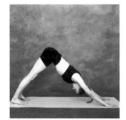

utktasana p96

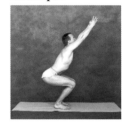

**adomukasvan-
asana p82**

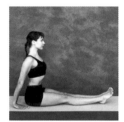

dandasana p40

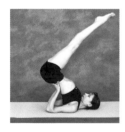

**ardasarvang-
asana p70**

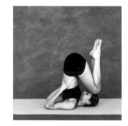

ardapindasana p44

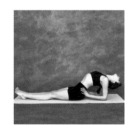

ardamatsyasana p72

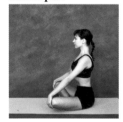

sukasana p24

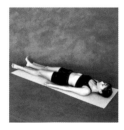

savasana p22

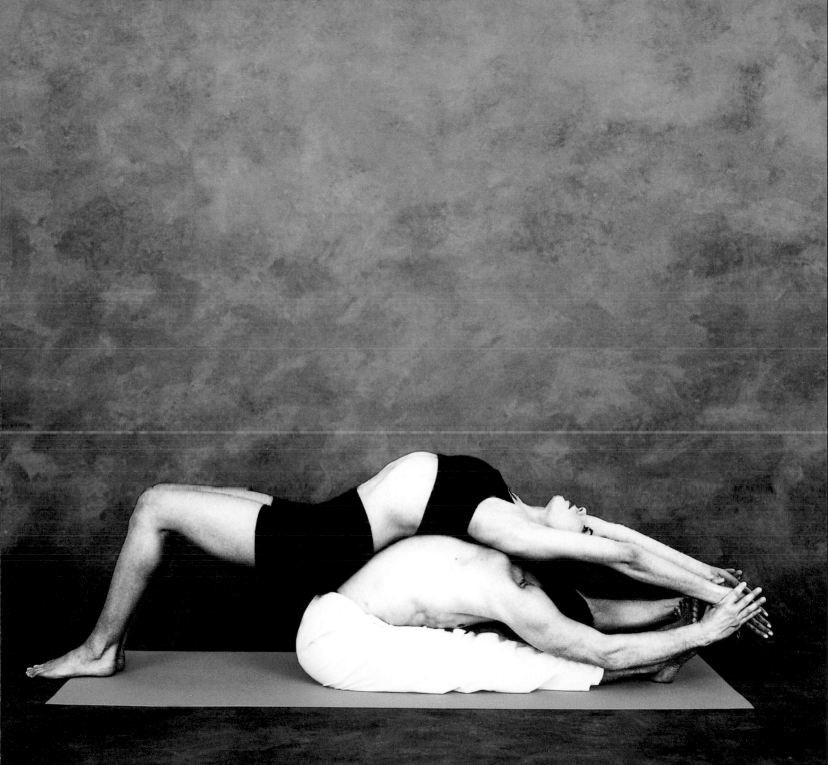

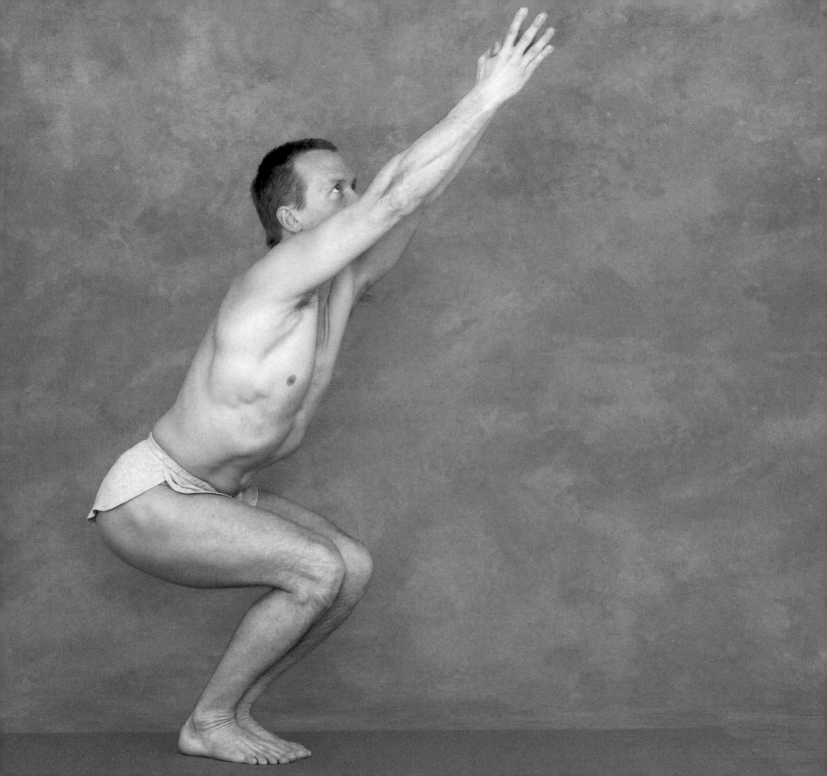

MOVING WITH THE BREATH

The breath is our link between body and mind. The activity of the body most directly and fluidly expressive of the mind is the breath. To transform our state of mind, the most simple and direct means is to change our breathing. The yoga postures automatically change our breathing by releasing tension from respiratory muscles and those that support them. The bandhas even more directly transform our breathing, and thereby the quality of our mind. But perhaps the most simple and accessible way of transforming the quality of the mind is by synchronizing the movement of the body with our breathing. This does not depend on large thoracic capacity, on flexibility, strength, or refined respiratory control.

The synchronization of movement with the breath is fundamental to yoga. It is known as vinyasa. Vinyasa is the basis of the sun salutations, the linked movements connecting postures and the steps that we take in and out of them. In vinyasa, any movement coincides exactly with either an inhalation or exhalation. The beginning of the inhale (or exhale) is also the beginning of the movement. The end of the inhale is the end of the movement. The speed of the body's movement also coincides exactly with the speed of the breath. A free inhalation and exhalation usually have a regular cycle. They begin picking up a little speed, then coast for most of their duration at a constant speed, then slow down towards the end. The exact nature and tempo of this cycle depends on the muscular and respiratory capacity. Allowing the body to follow this tempo as closely as possible is an important, subtle aspect of vinyasa. The more refined this synchronization, the more focused, alert and internalized the mind becomes. Vinyasa practice at this level triggers, through the rhythmic activity of the breath (pranayama), the profound meditative internalization known as pratyahara, the fifth limb of classical ashtanga yoga practice. Pratyahara then leads, with practice, directly to meditation.

In this lesson we focus on some movements that are the basis of the classical sun salutation. Being less demanding, they give more scope for refinement of the moving method of vinyasa, undisturbed by limitations of strength or flexibility. Each sequence is based on two or more body positions being connected into a flowing sequence based on the breath. Some of these positions are classical postures, some are intermediate steps into them. The key point in the practice of these sequences is not the postures, but the movement. They can be repeated as many times as you like. Whether or not exact synchronization occurs is not so important: looking for it is. When it eventually happens you will be rewarded with a taste of the therapeutic power of the meditative mind. In the beginning, just repeat the movements until you are well focused on what you are doing, without being distracted by external factors. Practice the combined group of sequences until you have opened your body up to its current capacity of movement. Then you can move into the yoga postures themselves to challenge and augment that capacity.

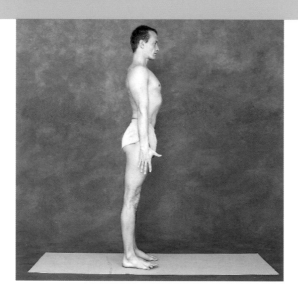

Standing pose is the basis of the first three dynamic sequences, as well as of many standing postures. It teaches and promotes full body awareness and integrity within a simple but challenging context. Standing pose immediately reveals our imbalances and limitations. It is important to be aware of what we have to compensate for, so we can adjust the emphasis of effort in our practice to foster balance and integrity in our body. It is especially in standing pose that we can take stock of the structural impact of our practice. Over the months and years we can notice changes in the way that we carry ourselves very easily in this posture, where nothing is demanded of us in terms of flexibility or strength that we might not have. Standing pose is the mirror in which we evaluate our condition and our practice. It can be used in practice for this purpose. Coming back to standing pose after a standing posture, we can settle into our physical presence, assimilating and feeling the impact of that posture before moving on to the next.

The external spirals of the feet (and legs) create grip in the outside of the pelvis, supporting the work of mulabandha, and offering stability. The internal spirals of the feet create openness and softness in the groins and pelvic floor, and support uddiyanabandha. Mulabandha stabilizes and supports the sacrum, diaphragm and lungs. Uddiyanabandha stabilizes the lower back and abdomen, opens the chest and lengthens the spine and core. This posture can also be done with the feet together.

urdvahastullola

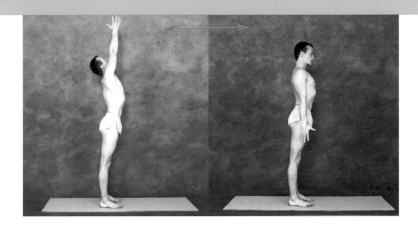

Urdvahastullola permits the cultivation of breath-body synchronization in an effortless context where only the arms and head are being moved. It is based on standing pose and its variation mountain pose.

utktullola

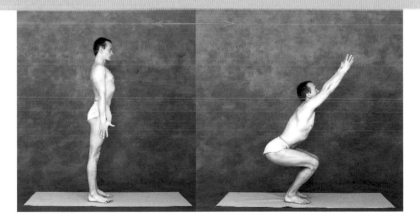

Utktullola challenges the cultivation of breath-body synchronization in a more demanding context where the movement of the legs engages the whole body. It is based on standing pose and the counterpose to standing-fold, fierce pose.

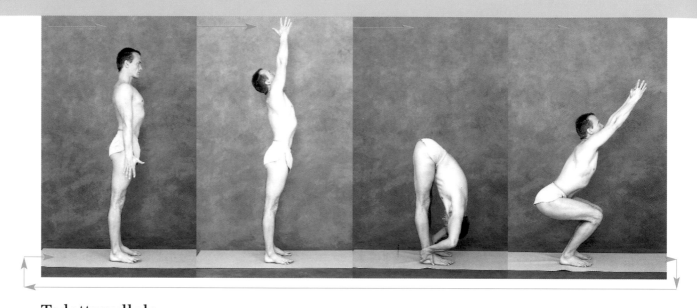

Tadottanullola challenges the cultivation of breath-body synchronization in a more demanding context. The four movements challenge stability, flexibility and strength. It is based on standing pose, mountain pose, standing-fold and fierce pose.

padottanullola

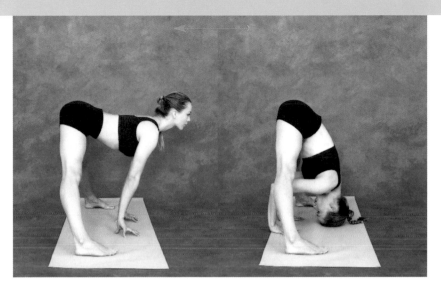

Padottanullola permits the cultivation of breath-body synchronization in the whole body, and is not too challenging. It is based on triangle pose, leg-stretch pose and its variation, gazing pose. Padottanullola can be varied by replacing gazing pose with triangle pose.

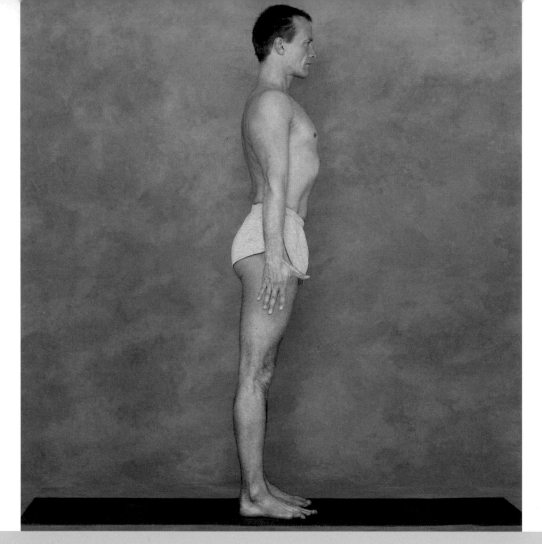

tadasana

This posture can be done with feet together or slightly apart. Vary this as part of your exploration of yoga. The legs are active and straight, as are the arms. The trunk is long, bandhas engaged, core soft. Shoulders are relaxed. Look ahead. Be careful not to strain the back by lifting aggressively. Also, do not overwork the legs by overemphasizing one or other of their spirals to compensate for your own imbalances. Be patient.

- Stand with your feet parallel and slightly apart.
- **Suck the thigh muscles into your thighbones so that your legs become straight and strong but not tense. Ground the four corners of each foot – ball of the big toe, ball of the little toe, inner heel and outer heel – evenly and fully.**
- Keeping both feet firmly grounded, internally spiral the feet and legs, pressing back from the ball of the big toe along the inner edge of the foot to the inner heel, then to the outer heel, in a rotating motion. Move the inner ankle bones back so that the groins move backwards, softening them, and move the inner edges of the knees outwards and broaden the pelvic floor.
- **Externally spiral the feet and legs. Press out from the ball of the big toe to the ball of the little toe, and lengthen the outer edge of the foot, pressing back from the ball of the little toe to the outer heel. Move the outer knees backwards, drawing the outer hips back at the same time.**
- Engaging the bandhas, broaden and flatten your pubic abdomen, keeping your anus soft. Lengthen your abdomen, sucking your solar plexus in so that the ribcrests activate and broaden. Keep your abdominal muscles passive, and place your hands on your hips.
- **Engage your hands, broadening the palms and lengthening the fingers as you spiral your arms by rolling the biceps out, while keeping the palms dynamically facing each other.**
- Raise your arms up alongside your ears, palms facing each other, arms spiralling and straight, shoulders relaxed. This is mountain pose. Hold for as long as you like, clarifying the activity of the bandhas, especially how they stabilize the pelvis, lengthen the lower back and open the chest.
- **Keeping your hands and arms engaged, lower them back to your sides, palms facing each other, shoulders relaxed.**

Hold the posture – feet and legs spiralling, bandhas engaged, aware of the free flow of inhalation and exhalation – until ready to release.

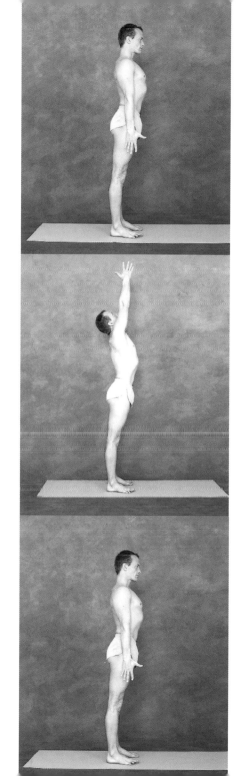

urdvahastullola

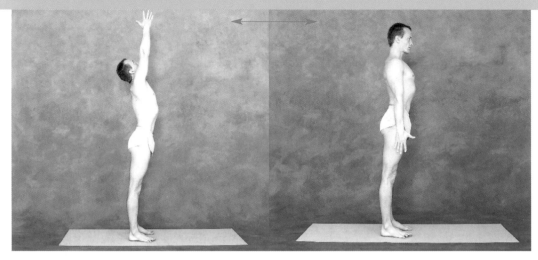

Repeat as many times as necessary.

utktullola

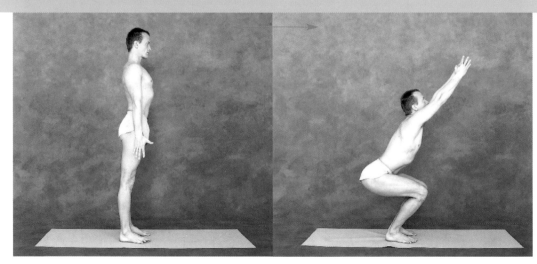

Repeat as many times as necessary.

tadottanullola

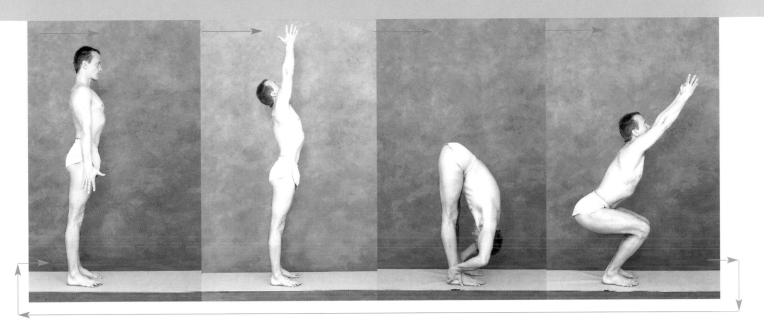

Repeat both exercises as many times as necessary.

padottanullola

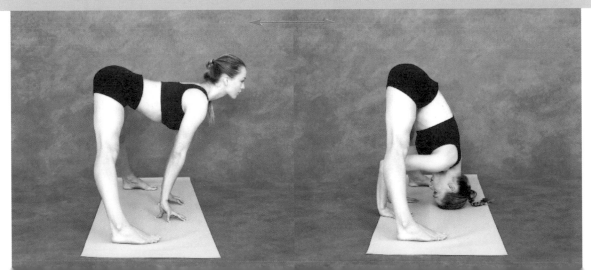

THE BREATH PRACTICE

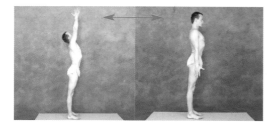

urdvahastullola p108

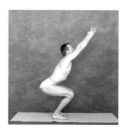

utktullola p108

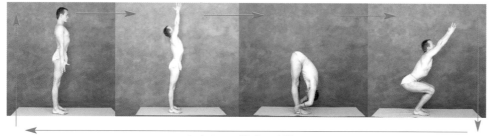

tadottanullola p109

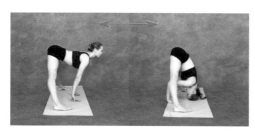

padottanullola p109

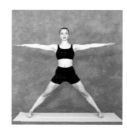

trikonasana p38

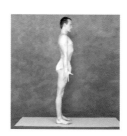

tadasana p106

utktasana p96

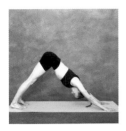 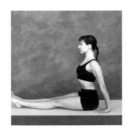 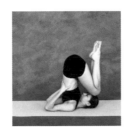 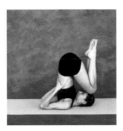 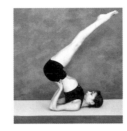

adomukasvanasana
p82

dandasana p40

ardapindasana p44

ardasarvangasana
p70

ardapindasana p44

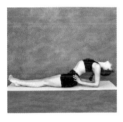 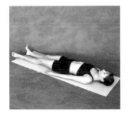 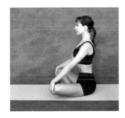

ardamatsyasana p72

savasana p22

sukasana p24

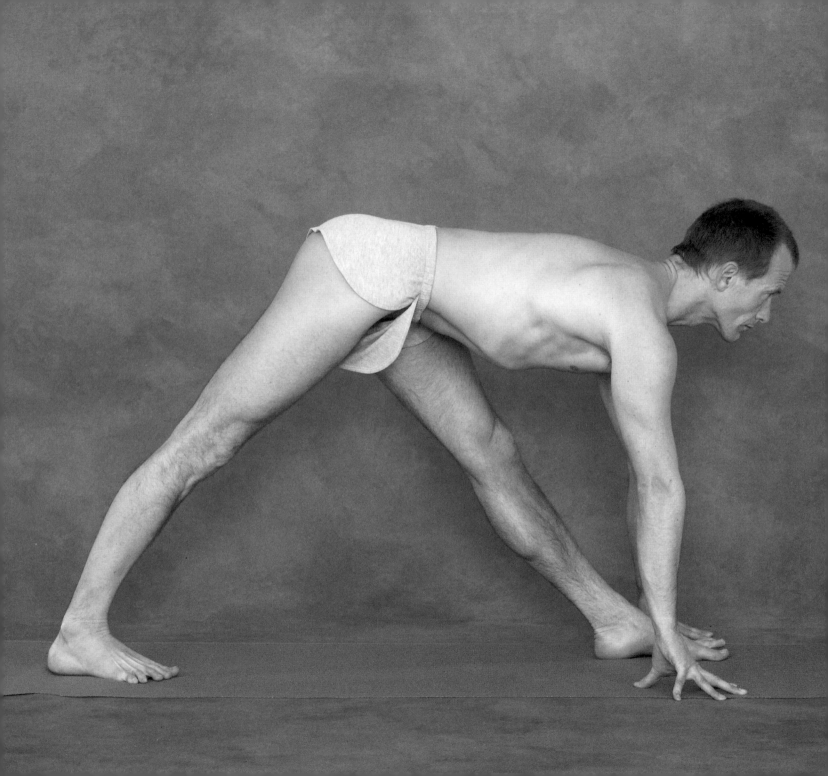

USING THE LEGS

When in standing postures, the work of the legs and the feet is to give stability and the possibility of comfort to the spine. The work is transmitted to the spine via the pelvis. The pelvis then becomes the main arena for the standing postures. The external spiral of the feet gathers energy and momentum inwards towards the centre from the periphery and creates the possibility of pelvic stability. The internal spiral releases energy and momentum outwards from the centre towards the periphery and creates the possibility of comfort. The external spiral creates firmness and cohesion. The internal spiral creates opening and softening. The external spiral supports mula bandha and provides protection to the sacrum and pelvis. The internal spiral supports uddiyana bandha and offers lift and opening to the trunk and lungs. These two poles of physical action must be balanced. When they balance each other, the pelvis works harmoniously – left balanced with right, top with bottom, back with front, centre with periphery, and inside with outside. This gives the spine the possibility of surrender.

Standing postures can be divided broadly into those based on standing pose and those based on triangle pose. It is especially those based on triangle pose that release and open the pelvis. This is a necessary prerequisite for free and full extension, rotation and flexion of the spine in forward bends, twists and backbends. Standing postures based on triangle pose can be divided into two main categories: those that turn the pelvis forwards and those that keep the pelvis rolled back. Both groups can be further divided into those with both legs straight and those with the front leg bent. In this lesson we focus on postures of both major groups, keeping both legs straight.

parsvasana

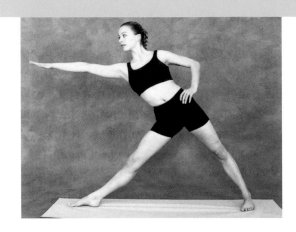

Reaching pose reveals the importance of the feet and legs to the pelvis and the spine. It teaches how to use the feet and legs to keep the weight even on the feet. This prevents hyperextension of the front leg by pushing the weight from the back heel to the ball of the front foot, and engaging the front thigh of the front leg correctly so that it pulls the thighbone forward out of the back of the knee. The reaching extension must come from the pelvis, not the waist. Do not bend at the waist. Rotate the pelvis. This rotation tends to make the back hip swing forward. It must, however, be kept rolled back.

Reaching pose develops the feet and legs, releases the spine and begins to open the hips and groins. It teaches how to keep the weight even on the feet. The external spiral of the front foot keeps the front leg centred and the buttock bone in line. The external spiral of the back foot keeps the back hip rolled back, and helps to transmit body weight forwards. The internal spirals of both feet (and legs) open the groins and pelvic floor and support the bandhas. Mulabandha gives stability to the pelvis, legs and the posture as a whole. Uddiyanabandha gives stability to the abdomen and lower back, length to the spine, breadth to the chest and openness to the posture as a whole.

parivritasana

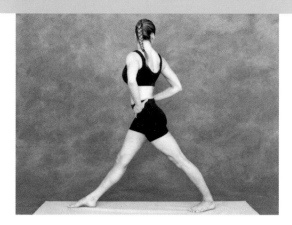

Twisting pose is a very simple but important posture, as it shows how easy it is to lose the activity of the feet and legs and leave the pelvis unsupported. By working from the spirals of the feet, through the spirals of the legs and into the pelvis, it teaches how to use the feet and legs to support, stabilize and open the pelvis. It also teaches how to keep the legs active when beginning to work in the trunk. It clarifies the effect of the internal spiral in particular. If this is not effectively activated, the groins collapse towards each other and the back and spine cannot release. The twisting action of the spine then becomes aggressive and instead of bringing softness to the back muscles, hardens them.

Twisting pose develops the feet and legs, softens the back and mobilizes the pelvis. The internal spiral of the front foot (and leg) keeps the groins supported and soft, and supports the extending rotation of the spine. The external spiral of the front foot will keep the pelvis on its vertical line. The internal spiral of the back foot helps to keep the leg straight and to support the back hip on its horizontal plane. The external spiral of the back foot stabilizes the pelvis and helps to transmit the weight forward to the front foot. Mulabandha gives stability to the pelvis, legs and the posture as a whole. Uddiyanabandha gives stability to the abdomen and lower back, length to the spine, breadth to the chest and openness to the posture as a whole.

salambatrikonasana

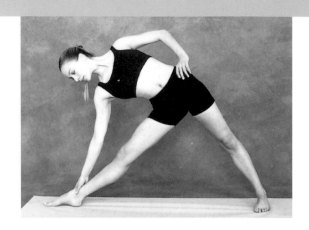

Supported triangle is a continuation of reaching pose, but it requires more work from the feet and legs to support the pelvis. They are then challenged more deeply to offer their support. If the feet and legs are not spiralling correctly this posture will create tension and discomfort in the back. There is a strong tendency to allow the back hip to roll forwards. Although this immediately makes the posture easier and more comfortable, it loses its ability to challenge tension in the hips, groins and sacrum. It is then reduced to a simple stretching exercise in which the hamstrings are likely to be overstretched and the lower waist to be compressed. This is not yoga. As with the reaching pose, there is a tendency for the front leg to hyperextend. Remember to keep the weight even between the feet by pressing forwards from the back heel, and to keep the front thigh muscles sucking into the bone.

Supported triangle releases the hips, groins and sacrum from tension. It develops the feet and legs, while releasing the spine. The external spiral of the front foot keeps the front leg centred and the buttock bone in line. The external spiral of the back foot keeps the back hip rolled back, and helps to transmit body weight forwards. The internal spirals of both feet (and legs) open the groins and pelvic floor and support the bandhas. Mulabandha gives stability to the pelvis, legs and the posture as a whole. Uddiyanabandha gives stability to the abdomen and lower back, length to the spine, breadth to the chest and openness to the posture as a whole.

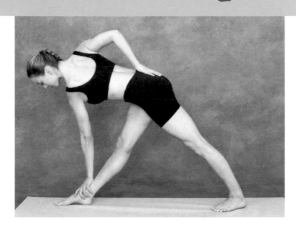

Revolving triangle

takes the work of twisting pose further. By extending the spine forward with the rotation, more work is imposed on the feet, legs and pelvis. They are then challenged more deeply to offer their support. If the feet and legs are not spiralling correctly this posture will create tension and discomfort in the back. It is also more likely to create hyperextension in the legs, if they stop working. It is vital to keep the weight even between the front and back foot. It tends to drop backwards to compensate for the forward movement of the spine. If this happens, push the weight forwards from the back foot to the ball of the front foot, spiralling both feet internally and externally.

Revolving triangle develops the feet and legs while mobilizing and strengthening the pelvis. It softens the back and releases the spine. The internal spiral of the front foot (and leg) will lift the front hip into its horizontal plane, and support the extending rotation of the spine. The external spiral of the front foot will take the pelvis into its vertical line. The internal spiral of the back foot helps to keep the leg straight and to support the back hip on its horizontal plane. The external spiral of the back foot stabilizes the pelvis and helps to transmit the weight forward to the front foot. Mulabandha gives stability to the pelvis, legs and the posture as a whole. Uddiyana-bandha gives stability to the abdomen and lower back, length to the spine, breadth to the chest and openness to the posture as a whole.

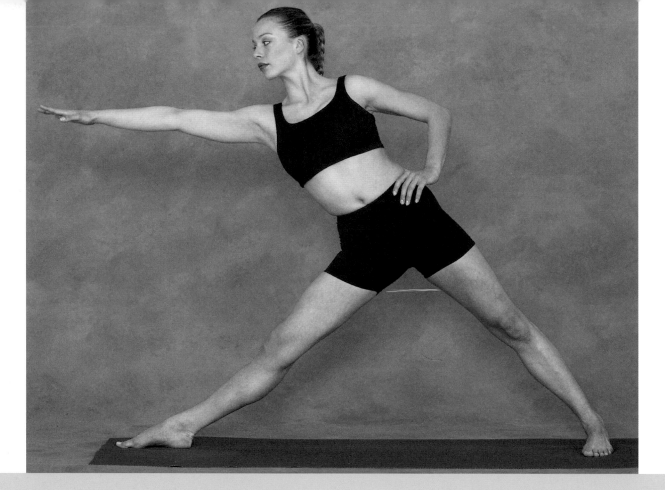

parsvasana

The weight is even between the front and back foot, between the heels and the balls of the feet and between the inner and outer edges of the feet. Feet are alive and spiralling, legs engaged and spiralling. Bandhas are engaged; shoulders relaxed; waist, trunk, spine and core long. Extend by rotating the pelvis, not bending the waist. Keep the inner and outer edges of both feet on the floor. Be accurate about the turn of the feet. The front foot is parallel to your mat, or turned 90 degrees from where the feet were parallel to each other. The back foot is turned in a little to create some opposition to rolling the back hip backwards from the external back foot spiral. As you become more open in the hips, the back foot will not need to be turned so much.

- Stand in hastatrikonasana with your hands on your hips.
- **Turn the right foot out exactly 90 degrees and the back foot in 10–15 degrees.**
- Roll the left hip back, broadening across the pubic bones.
- **Suck the thigh muscles into your thighbones so that your legs become straight and strong but not tense. Ground the four corners of each foot – ball of the big toe, ball of the little toe, inner heel and outer heel – evenly and fully.**
- Keeping both feet firmly grounded, internally spiral the feet and legs, pressing back from the ball of the big toe along the inner edge of the foot to the inner heel, then to the outer heel, in a rotating motion. Move the inner ankle bones back so that the groins move backwards, softening them and the buttocks. Move the inner edges of the knees outwards and broaden the pelvic floor.
- **Externally spiral the feet and legs, pressing out from the ball of the big toe to the ball of the little toe, and lengthening the outer edge of the foot, pressing back from the ball of the little toe to the outer heel. Move the outer knees backwards, drawing the outer hips back at the same time.**
- Engaging the bandhas, broaden and flatten your pubic abdomen, keeping your anus soft. Lengthen your abdomen, sucking your solar plexus in so that the ribcrests activate and broaden. Keep your abdominal muscles passive.
- **Keeping feet and legs spiralling, rotate the pelvis by dropping the right hip in and back towards the left groin, allowing the left hip to rotate upwards without dragging forwards.**
- Keeping your left hand on your hip, extend your right arm forwards as far as possible, lengthening your waist, trunk, spine and core.

Hold the posture – with feet, legs and bandhas maintaining the energetic and structural integrity of the posture; aware of the free flow of inhalation and exhalation; core soft – until ready to release. Repeat on the other side.

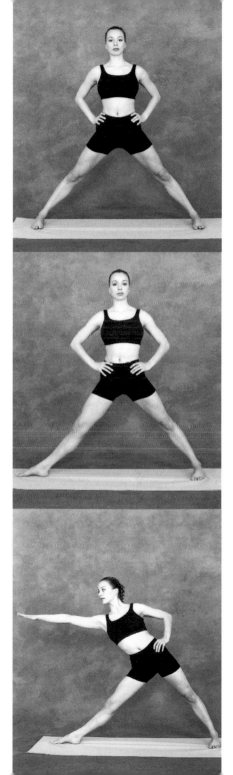

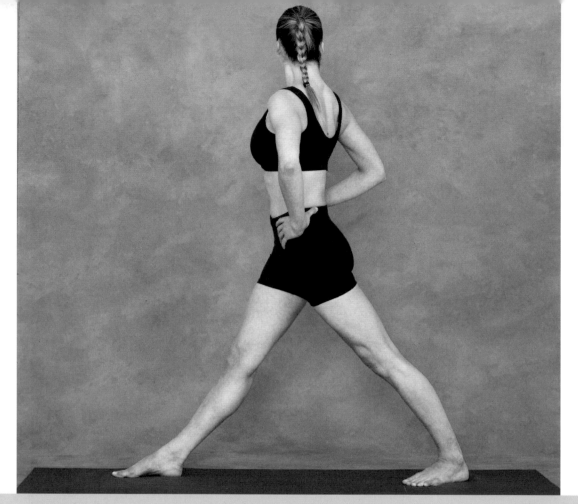

parivritasana

The weight is even between the front and back foot, between the heels and the balls of the feet and between the inner and outer edges of the feet. Feet are alive and spiralling, legs engaged and spiralling. Bandhas are engaged; shoulders relaxed; waist, trunk, spine and core long. Be careful not to force the twist and to cut the top of the trunk off from the bottom. Keep the inner and outer edges of both feet on the floor. Be accurate about the turn of the feet. The front foot is parallel to your mat, or turned 90 degrees from where the feet were parallel to each other. The back foot is turned well forwards to allow the back hip to come round in line with the front hip. As you become more open in the hips, the back foot will not need to be turned so much.

- Stand in hastatrikonasana with your hands on your hips.
- **Turn the right foot out exactly 90 degrees and the back foot in deeply enough to bring the back hip forward, in line with the front hip, including the whole trunk in the turn.**
- Lift the front of the pelvis upwards, keeping the spine vertical, chest lifted.
- **Suck the thigh muscles into your thighbones so that your legs become straight and strong but not tense. Ground the four corners of each foot – ball of the big toe, ball of the little toe, inner heel and outer heel – evenly and fully.**
- Keeping both feet firmly grounded, internally spiral the feet and legs, pressing back from the ball of the big toe along the inner edge of the foot to the inner heel, then to the outer heel, in a rotating motion. Move the inner ankle bones back so that the groins move backwards, softening them and the buttocks. Move the inner edges of the knees outwards and broaden the pelvic floor.
- **Externally spiral the feet and legs, pressing out from the ball of the big toe to the ball of the little toe, and lengthening the outer edge of the foot, pressing back from the ball of the little toe to the outer heel. Move the outer knees backwards, drawing the outer hips back at the same time.**
- Engaging the bandhas, broaden and flatten your pubic abdomen, keeping your anus soft. Lengthen your abdomen, sucking your solar plexus in so that the ribcrests activate and broaden. Keep your abdominal muscles passive.
- **Keeping feet and legs spiralling, roll the right shoulder back and look over it. Allow the whole trunk to rotate with this movement, keeping the pelvis up and in line, the groins supported and apart.**

Hold the posture – with feet, legs and bandhas maintaining the energetic and structural integrity of the posture; aware of the free flow of inhalation and exhalation; core soft – until ready to release. Repeat on the other side.

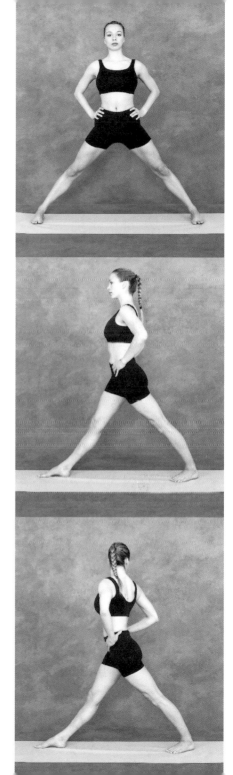

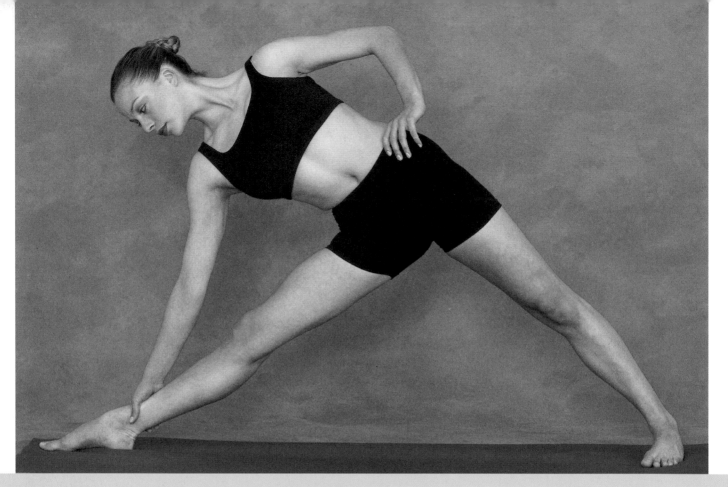

salambatrikonasana

- Stand in hastatrikonasana with your hands on your hips.
- **Turn the right foot out exactly 90 degrees and the back foot in deeply enough to bring the back hip forward in line with the front hip. Suck the thigh muscles into your thighbones so that your legs become straight and strong but not tense. Ground the four corners of each foot – ball of the big toe, ball of the little toe, inner heel and outer heel – evenly and fully.**
- Lift the front of the pelvis upwards, keeping the spine vertical and the chest lifted. Keeping both feet firmly grounded, internally spiral the feet and legs, pressing back from the ball of the big toe along the inner edge of the foot to the inner heel, then

to the outer heel, in a rotating motion. Move the inner ankle bones back so that the groins move backwards, softening them and the buttocks. Move the inner edges of the knees outwards and broaden the pelvic floor.

- **Externally spiral the feet and legs, pressing out from the ball of the big toe to the ball of the little toe, and lengthening the outer edge of the foot, pressing back from the ball of the little toe to the outer heel. Move the outer knees backwards, drawing the outer hips back at the same time.**
- Engaging the bandhas, broaden and flatten your pubic abdomen, keeping your anus soft. Lengthen your abdomen, sucking your solar plexus in so that the ribcrests activate and broaden. Keep your abdominal muscles passive.
- **Keeping feet and legs spiralling, pivot your pelvis forwards a little.**
- Extend your left arm forwards, lengthening your spine and trunk. Keep your right hand on your hip.
- **Take your left hand down onto your right shin or ankle by pivoting the pelvis until it is parallel to the floor.**
- Pressing with your left hand, turn your right armpit up towards the ceiling and look at your right foot.

Hold the posture – with feet, legs and bandhas maintaining the energetic and structural integrity of the posture; aware of the free flow of inhalation and exhalation; core soft – until ready to release. Repeat on the other side.

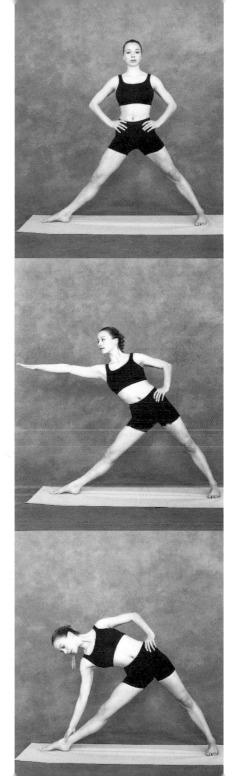

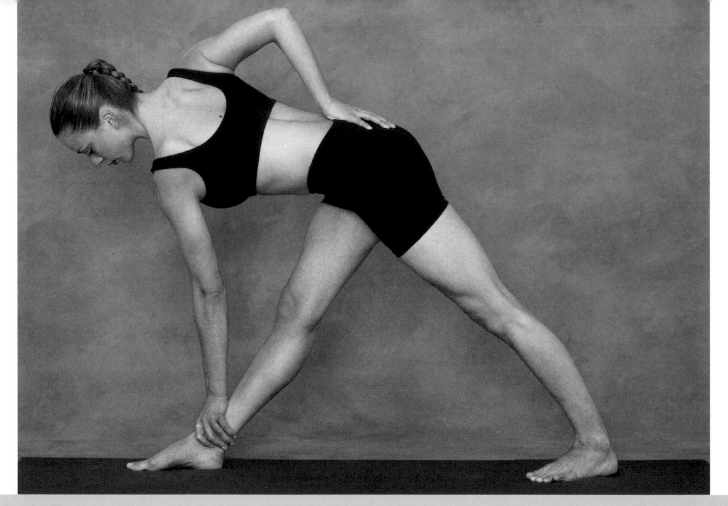

salambaparivritatrikonasana

The weight is even between the front and back foot, between the heels and the balls of the feet and between the inner and outer edges of the feet. Feet are alive and spiralling, legs engaged and spiralling. Bandhas are engaged; shoulders relaxed; waist, trunk, spine and core long. Be careful not to force the twist and to cut the top of the trunk off from the bottom. Keep the inner and outer edges of both feet on the floor. Be accurate about the turn of the feet. The front foot is parallel to your mat, or turned 90 degrees from where the feet were parallel to each other. The back foot is turned well forwards to allow the back hip to come round in line with the front hip. As you become more open in the hips, the back foot will not need to be turned so much.

- Stand in hastatrikonasana with your hands on your hips.
- **Turn the right foot out exactly 90 degrees and the back foot in deeply enough to bring the back hip forward in line with the front hip. Suck the thigh muscles into your thighbones so that your legs become straight and strong but not tense. Ground the four corners of each foot – ball of the big toe, ball of the little toe, inner heel and outer heel – evenly and fully.**
- Lift the front of the pelvis upwards, keeping the spine vertical and the chest lifted. Keeping both feet firmly grounded, internally spiral the feet and legs, pressing back from the ball of the big toe along the inner edge of the foot to the inner heel, then to the outer heel, in a rotating motion. Move the inner ankle bones back so that the groins move backwards, softening them and the buttocks. Move the inner edges of the knees outwards and broaden the pelvic floor.
- **Externally spiral the feet and legs, pressing out from the ball of the big toe to the ball of the little toe, and lengthening the outer edge of the foot, pressing back from the ball of the little toe to the outer heel. Move the outer knees backwards, drawing the outer hips back at the same time.**
- Engaging the bandhas, broaden and flatten your pubic abdomen, keeping your anus soft. Lengthen your abdomen, sucking your solar plexus in so that the ribcrests activate and broaden. Keep your abdominal muscles passive.
- **Keeping feet and legs spiralling, pivot your pelvis forwards a little.**
- Extend your left arm forwards, lengthening your spine and trunk. Keep your right hand on your hip.
- **Take your left hand down onto your right shin or ankle by pivoting the pelvis until it is parallel to the floor.**
- Pressing with your left hand, turn your right armpit up towards the ceiling and look at your right foot.

Hold the posture – with feet, legs and bandhas maintaining the energetic and structural integrity of the posture; aware of the free flow of inhalation and exhalation; core soft – until ready to release. Repeat on the other side.

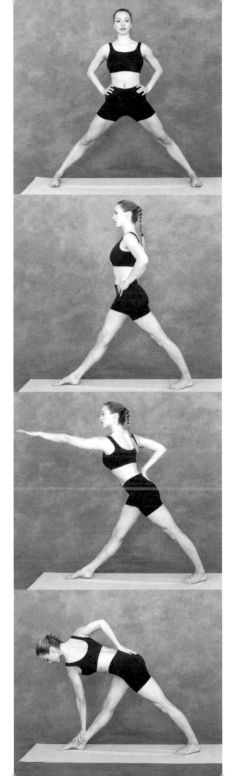

THE STANDING PRACTICE

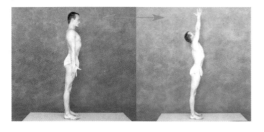

urdvahastullola p108

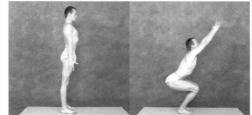

utktullola p108

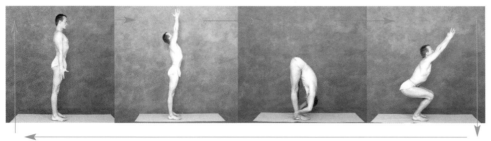

tadottanullola p109

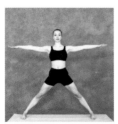

trikonasana p38

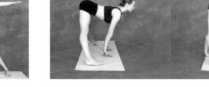

padottanullola p109

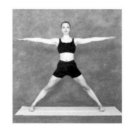

trikonasana p38

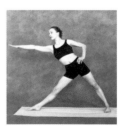

parsvasana p118

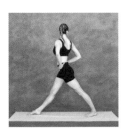 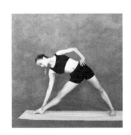 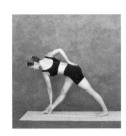 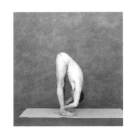 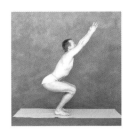

parivritasana p120 salambatrikon- salambaparivrita- uttanasana p96 utktasana p96
asana p122 trikonasana p124

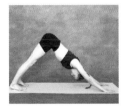 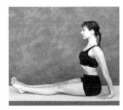 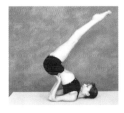 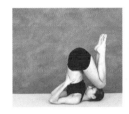 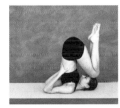

adomukasvan- dandasana p40 ardapindasana p44 ardasarvang- ardapindasana p44
asana p82 asana p70

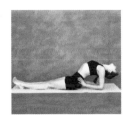 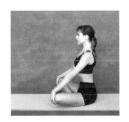 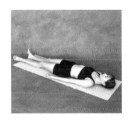

ardamatsyasana savasana p22 sukasana p24
p72

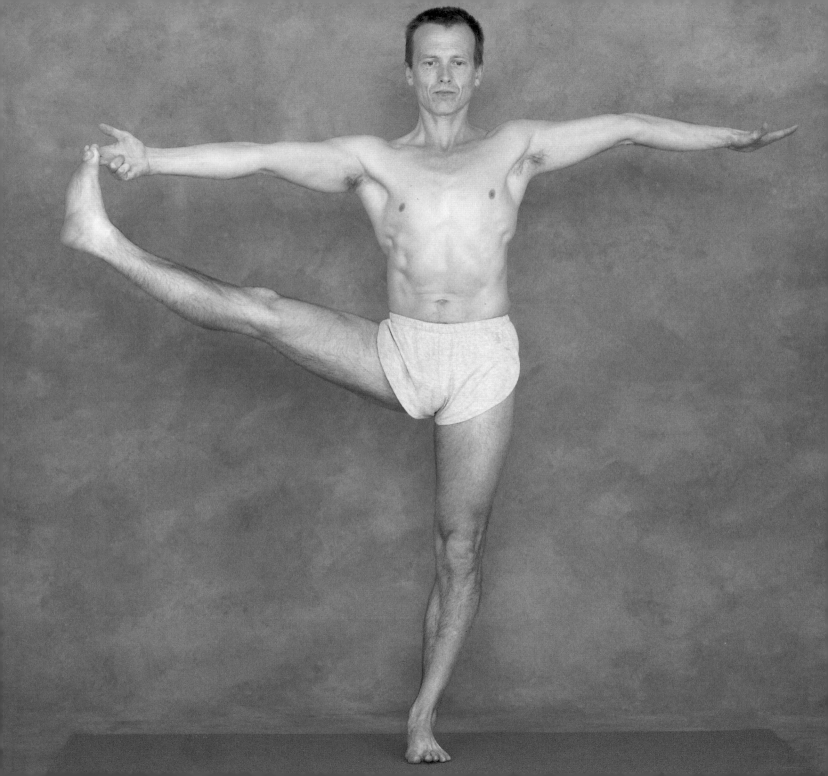

ADJUSTING THE PELVIS SIDEWAYS

In this lesson we will focus on three standing postures based on reaching pose, all having the pelvis rolled back and the front leg bent. They all have a similar use of the feet, legs and pelvis, and are directly related to reaching pose and supported triangle. In all five cases the dynamic of the pelvis is the same. This involves keeping the back hip rolled back, so that the pelvis stays in line when the feet are turned forward. This keeps the posture on a single plane. The line of the pelvis is, of course, established and maintained by the activity of the legs, which in turn depends entirely on the position and spirallic activity of the feet.

To prevent the back hip rolling forward, emphasis needs to be given to the external spiral of the back foot. This is transmitted up the leg and into the pelvis, keeping the hip rolled back. If the back leg is not straight there will be no spirallic transmission to the pelvis, and the hip will roll forward. The front knee must make an exact right angle. The line of the knee also depends on the position of the front buttock bone. It must be kept in, by rotating or spiralling it towards the navel from the grounding action of the external spiral of the front foot. When you have a right angle the thighbone is parallel to the floor, the shinbone is perpendicular and the knee is directly above the heel. The leg is bent by lowering the head of the thighbone down to the height of the knee. This automatically takes the knee forwards and brings the trunk and pelvis down. This downwards movement should not be prevented but it should be resisted. This is done by moving the hip sockets upwards in a strong spirallic motion that also takes the hip socket inwards and upwards towards the navel and keeps the buttock bone in line. There is then a strong opposition between the lowering of the thighbone and the spiralling lift of the hip socket. To keep half your weight on the back foot, press to the heel of the back foot from the heel of the front. The weight must be kept even across each foot by emphasizing the inner edge of the front foot and the outer edge of the back foot. The external spiral of the front foot keeps the front buttock bone in line, and spiralling in and up towards the navel. The external spiral of the back foot keeps the back hip rolled back, and the hip socket spiralling towards the navel. The internal spiral of the front foot softens the groin and broadens the pelvic floor. The internal spiral of the back foot softens the groin, broadens the pelvic floor and keeps the buttock soft. Mulabandha gives stability to the pelvis, legs and the posture as a whole. Uddiyanabandha gives stability to the abdomen and lower back, length to the spine, breadth to the chest and openness to the posture as a whole.

Mastering these postures does not require great flexibility, or strength. It is a question of awareness and resolve. Because they are done standing they can be tiring when the body is not open enough to do them fully. It is vital in hatha yoga to distinguish clearly between postures 'done fully' and postures 'done in the correct manner'. Hatha yoga is not about imposing on yourself. It is not about trying to force your body into the predetermined shape of specific postures. It is about opening your body so that it naturally and effortlessly accommodates the postures.

A posture can only be done 'fully' when each part of the body involved is completely free from tension, and has sufficient strength. This is not always going to be possible, especially in the beginning. It may never be possible. What is important is that you are doing the postures in the correct manner. This means doing them so that they release the tension that is inhibiting the posture, develop the strength the posture demands, and awaken the intelligence that the posture requires. The key to this is intelligent application of the three principles: the foundation, the core and the dynamic of the bandhas. Intelligent application of these principles means applying them with sensitivity, honesty, openness, focus, generosity, commitment, contentment, passion, self-reflection and devotion. By approaching the postures in this way they will open the body. As the body opens the postures will become easier and easier.

A posture well done cannot be measured by a protractor and compass. It is a measure of the judicious and dedicated application of the resources you have available: the flexibility that you have in this moment; the strength that you have in this moment; the energy that you have in this moment; your attentiveness; your intent. A beginner student mobilising all their resources while only half way into a posture is getting exactly as much from the posture as an advanced student mobilising all their resources to be fully in the posture. And much more than a flexible student who is in the full pose without mobilising all their resources. You are doing a posture well when you are doing it to the best of your ability. Then it will be challenging you. Then it will be opening you. Then it will be developing you.

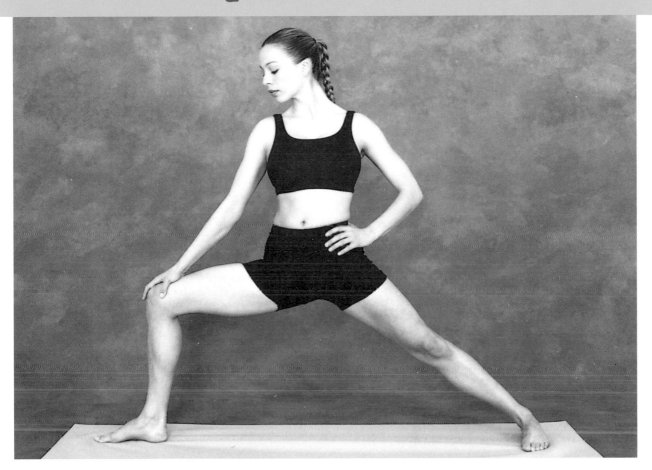

Supported side warrior teaches the correct line of the front leg and the correct feet spacing for all of these postures. It develops the feet and legs and opens the groins while mobilizing and strengthening the pelvis. It softens the back and releases the spine. It teaches how to keep the weight even on the feet. The external spiral of the front foot keeps the front leg centred and the buttock bone in line. The external spiral of the back foot keeps the back hip rolled back. The internal spirals of both feet (and legs) open the groins and pelvic floor and support the bandhas. Mulabandha gives stability to the pelvis, legs and the posture as a whole. Uddiyanabandha gives stability to the abdomen and lower back, length to the spine, breadth to the chest and openness to the posture as a whole.

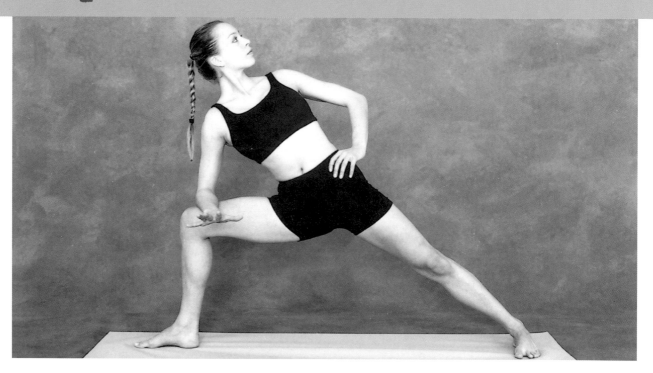

Supported lunge teaches the correct line of both the back hip and the front buttock bone. The back hip is supported from the external spiral of the back foot. The front buttock bone must be kept tucked in towards the perineum, and is supported from the external spiral of the front foot. Use the internal spirals of the feet to keep the groins soft and back.

Supported lunge develops the feet and legs while mobilizing and strengthening the pelvis. It opens the pelvis, softens the back and releases the spine. It teaches how to keep the weight even on the feet. The external spiral of the front foot keeps the front leg centred and the buttock bone in line. The external spiral of the back foot keeps the back hip rolled back, and helps to transmit body weight forwards. The internal spirals of both feet (and legs) open the groins and pelvic floor and support the bandhas. Mulabandha gives stability to the pelvis, legs and the posture as a whole. Uddiyanabandha gives stability to the abdomen and lower back, length to the spine, breadth to the chest and openness to the posture as a whole.

parsvavirabadrasana

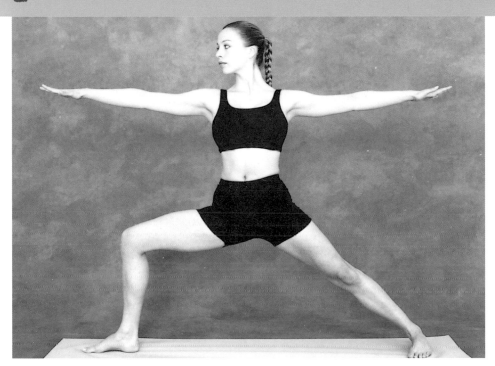

Side warrior teaches how to transmit the work of the feet and legs into the upper body so that the trunk, spine and core lengthen and the chest lifts and opens. The arms spiral out of the armpits parallel to the floor, armpits directly above their hipbones.

It develops the arms, feet and legs while mobilizing and strengthening the pelvis. It opens the pelvis, softens the back and releases the spine. It teaches how to keep the weight even on the feet. The external spiral of the front foot keeps the front leg centred and the buttock bone in line. The external spiral of the back foot keeps the back hip rolled back, and helps to transmit body weight forwards. The internal spirals of both feet (and legs) open the groins and pelvic floor and support the bandhas. Mulabandha gives stability to the pelvis, legs and the posture as a whole. Uddiyanabandha gives stability to the abdomen and lower back, length to the spine, breadth to the chest and openness to the posture as a whole.

This pose can be done dynamically following the principles outlined in Lesson Seven.

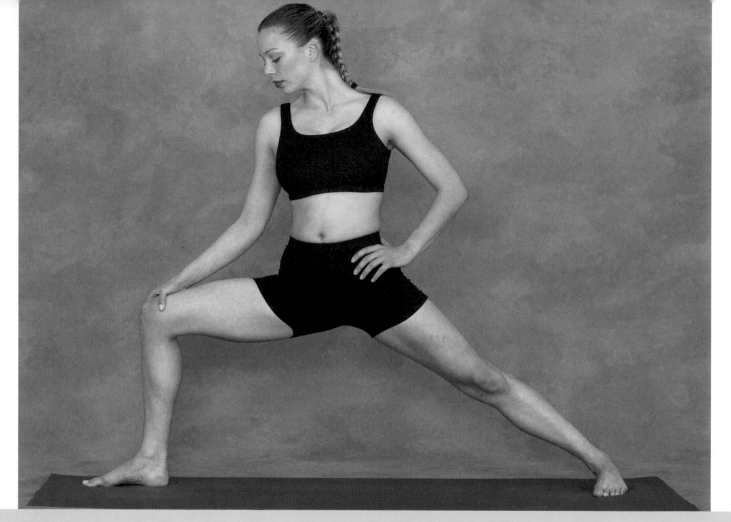

salambaparsvavirabadrasana

The feet are carefully positioned so that when the front leg is bent you have a true right angle at the knee. The knee is directly above the heel, the thighbone is parallel to the floor, the shinbone perpendicular. The weight is even between the front and back foot, between the heels and the balls of the feet and between the inner and outer edges of the feet. The front buttock bone is kept tucked in by the right foot. The back hip is kept rolled back by the back foot. Use the front hand and arm to keep the trunk vertical and long, and maintain the line of the front leg and knee. Keep the shoulders relaxed.

- Stand in hastatrikonasana, feet parallel, hands on hips.
- **Turn the right foot out exactly 90 degrees and the back foot in 10–15 degrees.**
- Roll the left hip back, broadening across the pubic bones.
- **Suck the thigh muscles into your thighbones so that your legs become straight and strong but not tense. Ground the four corners of each foot – ball of the big toe, ball of the little toe, inner heel and outer heel – evenly and fully, and engage the internal and external spirals of both feet and legs.**
- Engaging the bandhas, broaden and flatten your pubic abdomen, keeping your anus and core soft. Lengthen your abdomen, sucking your solar plexus in so that the ribcrests activate and broaden. Keep your abdominal muscles passive.
- **Keeping your weight even on your feet, and the left leg straight and spiralling from the foot, bend your right leg until you have a perfect right angle at the knee.**
- Extend your right arm forwards and place your hand on the right thigh by the knee.
- **Pressing with your right hand, make your trunk and spine vertical.**

Hold the posture – with feet, legs and bandhas maintaining the energetic and structural integrity of the posture; aware of the free flow of inhalation and exhalation; core soft – until ready to release. Repeat on the other side.

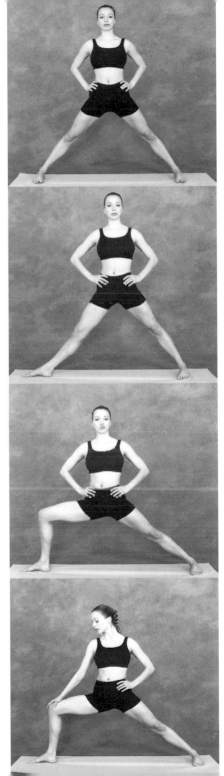

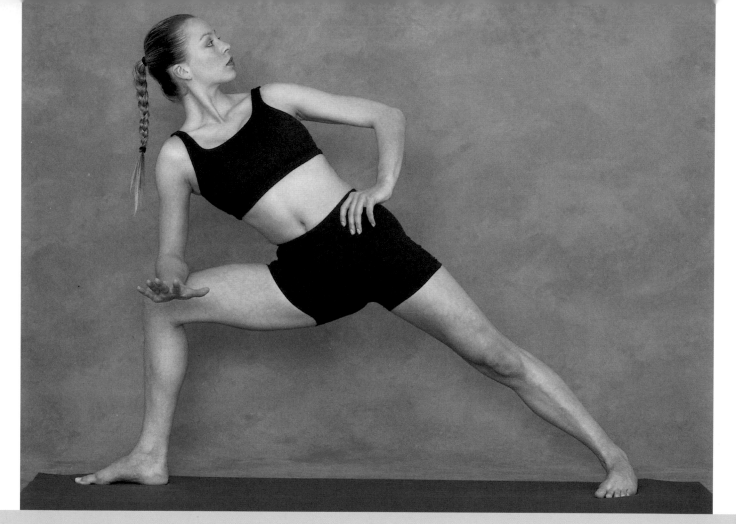

salambaparsvakonasana

The feet are carefully positioned, so that when the front leg is bent you have a true right angle at the knee. The knee is directly above the heel, the thighbone is parallel to the floor, the shinbone perpendicular. The weight is even between the front and back foot, between the heels and the balls of the feet and between the inner and outer edges of the feet. The front buttock bone is kept tucked in by the right foot. The back hip is kept rolled back by the back foot. Use the front arm to keep the trunk long, and maintain the line of the front leg and knee. Keep the shoulders relaxed.

- Stand in hastatrikonasana with your hands on your hips.
- **Turn the right foot out exactly 90 degrees and the back foot in 10–15 degrees.**
- Roll the left hip back, broadening across the pubic bones.
- **Suck the thigh muscles into your thighbones so that your legs become straight and strong but not tense. Ground the four corners of each foot – ball of the big toe, ball of the little toe, inner heel and outer heel – evenly and fully, and engage the internal and external spirals of both feet and legs.**
- Engaging the bandhas, broaden and flatten your pubic abdomen, keeping your anus and core soft. Lengthen your abdomen, sucking your solar plexus in so that the ribcrests activate and broaden. Keep your abdominal muscles passive.
- **Keeping your weight even on your feet, and the left leg straight and spiralling from the foot, bend your right leg until you have a perfect right angle at the knee.**
- Extend your right arm forwards until the armpit is above the knee and the right side of your trunk is extending at an angle to the floor.
- **Bending your right arm, place the elbow on the thigh, keeping the hand open.**
- Pressing your elbow onto your thigh, turn the left armpit towards the ceiling and look over your left shoulder.

Hold the posture – with feet, legs and bandhas maintaining the energetic and structural integrity of the posture; aware of the free flow of inhalation and exhalation; core soft – until ready to release. Repeat on the other side.

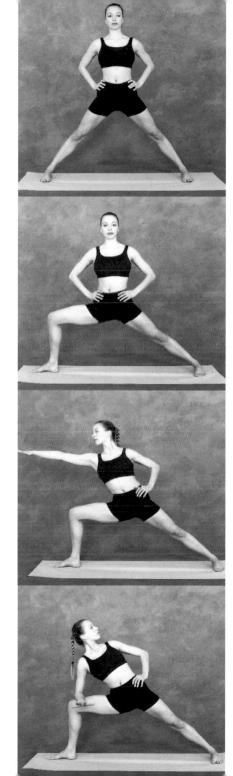

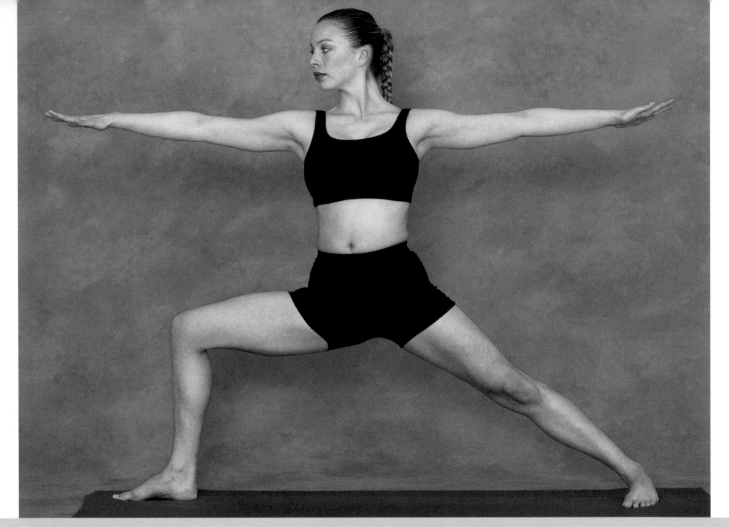

parsvavirabadrasana

The feet are carefully positioned, so that when the front leg is bent you have a true right angle at the knee. The knee is directly above the heel, the thighbone is parallel to the floor, the shinbone perpendicular. The weight is even between the front and back foot, between the heels and the balls of the feet and between the inner and outer edges of the feet. The front buttock bone is kept tucked in by the right foot. The back hip is kept rolled back by the back foot. Use the arms to open the chest. Keep the shoulders relaxed. The armpits are kept directly above their hipbones, arms spiralling parallel to the floor.

- Stand in trikonasana, feet parallel, arms spiralling parallel to the floor.
- **Turn the right foot out exactly 90 degrees and the back foot in 10–15 degrees.**
- Roll the left hip back, broadening across the pubic bones and look along the right arm.
- **Suck the thigh muscles into your thighbones so that your legs become straight and strong but not tense. Ground the four corners of each foot – ball of the big toe, ball of the little toe, inner heel and outer heel – evenly and fully, and engage the internal and external spirals of both feet and legs.**
- Engaging the bandhas, broaden and flatten your pubic abdomen, keeping your anus and core soft. Lengthen your abdomen, sucking your solar plexus in so that the ribcrests activate and broaden. Keep your abdominal muscles passive.
- **Keeping your weight even on your feet, and the left leg straight and spiralling from the foot, bend your right leg until you have a perfect right angle at the knee.**

Hold the posture – with feet, legs and bandhas maintaining the energetic and structural integrity of the posture; aware of the free flow of inhalation and exhalation; core soft – until ready to release. Repeat on the other side.

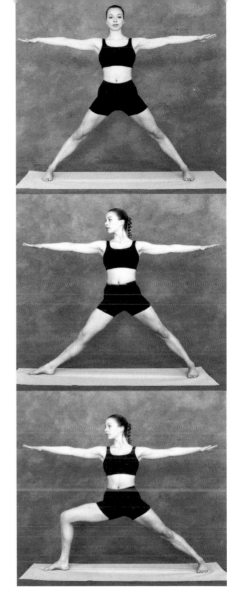

THE LUNGE PRACTICE

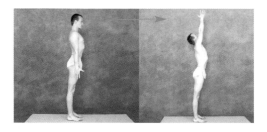

urdvahastullola p108

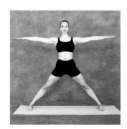

utktullola p108

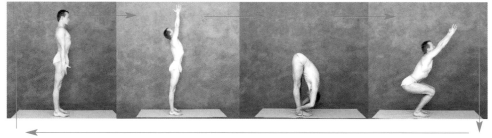

tadottanullola p109

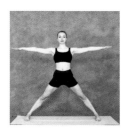

trikonasana p38

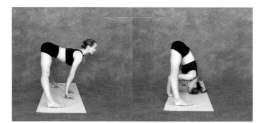

padottanullola p109

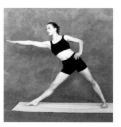

trikonasana p38

parsvasana p118

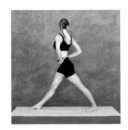 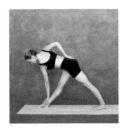 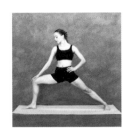 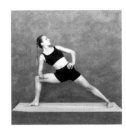 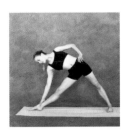

parivritasana p120 salambatrikon-asana p122 salambaparivrita-trikonasana p124 salambaparsvavira-badrasana p134 salambaparsvakon-asana p136

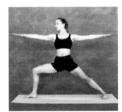 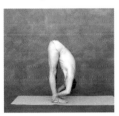 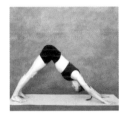 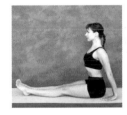 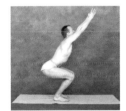

parsvavirabadr-asana p138 uttanasana p96 utktasana p96 adomukasvan-asana p82 dandasana p40

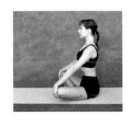 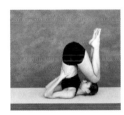 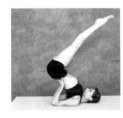 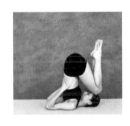 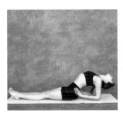

sukasana p24 ardapindasana p44 ardasarvangasana p70 ardapindasana p44 ardamatsyasana p72

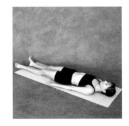

savasana p22 sukasana p24

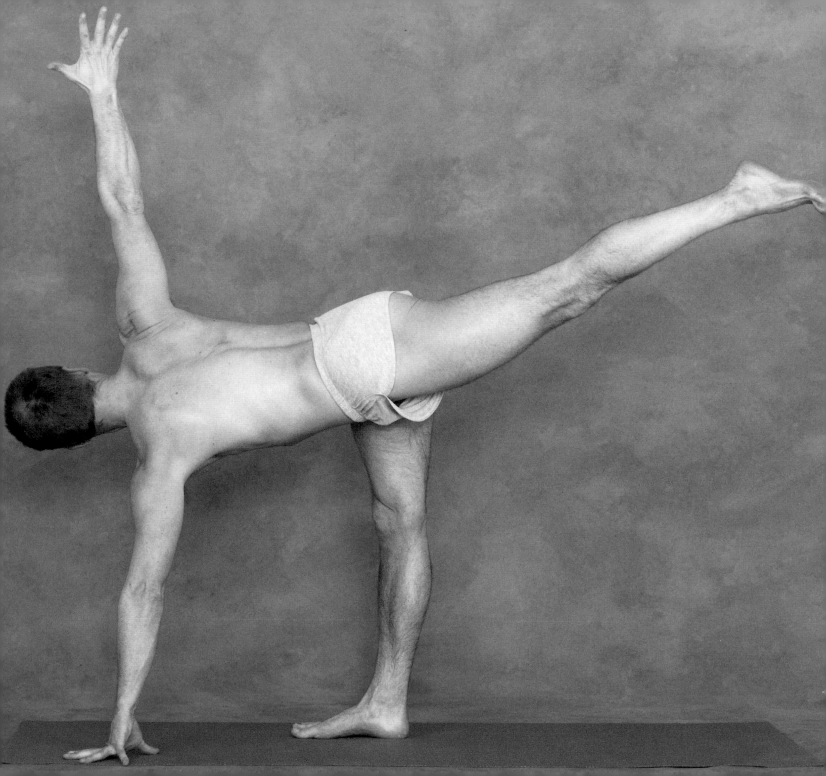

ADJUSTING THE PELVIS FORWARDS

These postures are strenuous for many people. Be willing to release them if you cannot become stable. If you find you are shaking, and that grounding your feet and working your legs does not release it, you may be too tired to get any benefit from these postures. Try tomorrow.

In this lesson we will focus on three standing postures based on triangle pose, all having the pelvis turned forwards and the front leg bent. They all have a similar use of the feet, legs and pelvis. These postures are directly related to twisting pose and revolving triangle. In all five cases the dynamic of the pelvis is the same. This involves bringing the back hip forwards, so that the pelvis dissects the line of the legs when the feet are turned forward. This establishes the posture on two planes. This is not easy for most people to do. Tightness in the legs, groins and hips prevents a full rotation of the pelvis. The more you turn your back foot in, the easier you will find it. If you find the front foot cannot ground the inner edge, move the foot slightly further out to the side until it becomes possible to ground the inner and outer edges of the feet equally. Only do this just as much as you need or you will lose the centre of the posture. Again, make sure you have a true right angle and that the front groin does not collapse. The feet must be spaced accurately, and the front leg must be bent the correct amount and in the correct manner. The front buttock bone must again be kept in from the external spiral of the front foot.

Be especially vigilant of the back leg. Because of the difficulty of bringing the pelvis forwards, it is easy to lose the support of the back foot. The reason for this is that when it turns in to allow the pelvis to turn, the inner leg is asked to lengthen more to keep the foot grounded. If the foot does not remain grounded then it is almost impossible to keep the leg straight. Too much weight and work then falls on the front leg, which can easily tire and strain. At the same time, the pelvis will be uneven, rendering the trunk and spine uneven too. This can distort and strain the lower back. You therefore have to find a trade-off between turning the foot more to allow forward movement of the hip, and turning it less to keep it grounded. This ongoing process is a lesson in the art of opposition in hatha yoga. Keeping the integrity of the back leg comes from the internal spiral of the foot. This transmits through the leg and takes the inner knee and the groin back. This, at the same time, brings the back hip more forwards.

All the adjustments that you make are limited by others. This opposition prevents excess movement in one direction or plane. Any spirallic adjustment is balanced by others, but usually there are one or two primary ones. As you go deeper into your practice these relationships will express themselves even if you do not become conceptually conscious of them. This process of structural opposition is a manifestation of the internal dynamic of the bandhas.

The external spiral of the front foot keeps the front buttock bone in line and spiralling in and up towards the navel. The external spiral of the back foot supports the hip and keeps the trunk even. The internal spiral of the front foot softens the groin and broadens the pelvic floor. The internal spiral of the back foot softens the groin, broadens the pelvic floor, keeps the buttock soft and supports the back leg and the spine. Mulabandha gives stability to the pelvis, legs and the posture as a whole. Uddiyanabandha gives stability to the abdomen and lower back, length to the spine, breadth to the chest and openness to the posture as a whole.

salambavirabadrasana

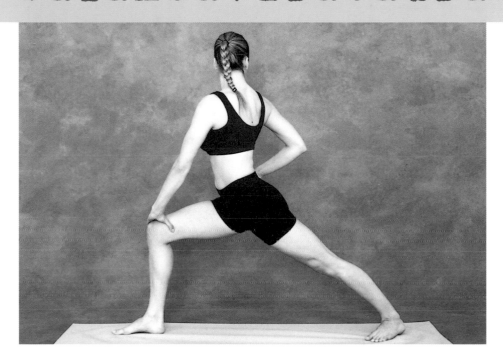

Supported warrior teaches the correct line of the front leg, and the lift of the pelvis. The pelvis tends to drop towards the front thigh. This not only puts pressure and strain on the lower back, but collapses the chest, inhibiting the breath. Use the front hand to resist this tendency, learning to lift the pelvis at the same time that you turn it.

Supported warrior develops the feet and legs, softens the back and mobilizes the pelvis. The internal spiral of the front foot (and leg) keeps the groins supported and soft, and supports the extending rotation of the spine. The external spiral of the front foot will keep the pelvis on its vertical line. The internal spiral of the back foot helps to keep the leg straight and to support the back hip on its horizontal plane. The external spiral of the back foot stabilizes the pelvis. Mulabandha gives stability to the pelvis, legs and the posture as a whole. Uddiyana-bandha gives stability to the abdomen and lower back, length to the spine, breadth to the chest and openness to the posture as a whole.

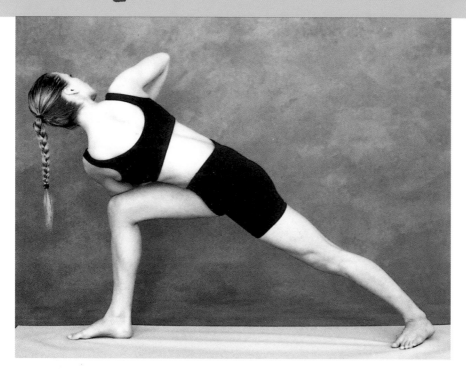

Lunging salute is a supported twist. It teaches how to support the rotation of the spine from the internal spiral of the back foot. Because of the forward extension of the trunk there is no need to keep the hips lifted as they turn.

Lunging salute develops the feet and legs, softens the back and mobilizes the pelvis. It releases and nourishes the vertebrae, establishing and maintaining mobility in the spinal column. The internal spiral of the front foot (and leg) keeps the groins supported and soft, and supports the extending rotation of the spine. The external spiral of the front foot will keep the pelvis on its vertical line. The internal spiral of the back foot helps to keep the leg straight and to support the back groin. The external spiral of the back foot stabilizes the pelvis. Mulabandha gives stability to the pelvis, legs and the posture as a whole. Uddiyanabandha gives stability to the abdomen and lower back, length to the spine, breadth to the chest and openness to the posture as a whole.

hastavirabadrasana

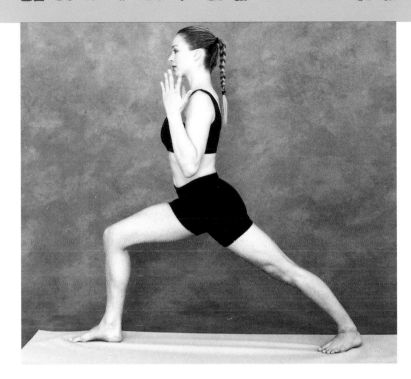

Warrior pose teaches how to transmit the work of the feet and legs into the upper body so that the trunk, spine and core lengthen and the chest lifts and opens, while the pelvis remains vertical and stable.

Warrior pose develops the feet and legs, softens the back and mobilizes the pelvis. It also opens the chest and mobilizes the top spine. The internal spiral of the front foot (and leg) keeps the groins supported and soft, and supports the extending rotation of the spine. The external spiral of the front foot will keep the pelvis on its vertical line. The internal spiral of the back foot helps to keep the leg straight and to turn the pelvis. The external spiral of the back foot stabilizes the pelvis. Mulabandha gives stability to the pelvis, legs and the posture as a whole. Uddiyanabandha gives stability to the abdomen and lower back, length to the spine, breadth to the chest and openness to the posture as a whole.

This pose can be done dynamically as in the method learned in Lesson Seven.

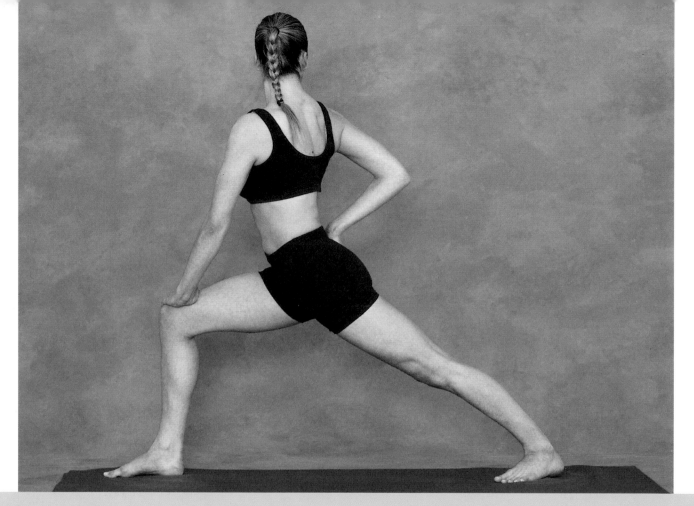

salambavirabadrasana

The feet are separated exactly so that when the front leg is bent you have a true right angle at the knee. The knee is directly above the heel, the thighbone is parallel to the floor, the shinbone perpendicular. The weight is even between the front and back foot, between the heels and the balls of the feet and between the inner and outer edges of the feet. The front buttock bone is kept tucked in by the front foot external spiral. The back leg is kept straight from the back foot internal spiral. The pelvis is kept in line from the back foot internal spiral. The pelvis is kept up from the grounding of the front foot. Use the front hand and arm to keep the trunk vertical and long and to maintain the line of the front leg and knee. Keep the shoulders relaxed.

- Stand in hastatrikonasana with your hands on your hips.
- **Turn the right foot out exactly 90 degrees and the back foot in deeply enough to bring the back hip forward in line with the front hip. Suck the thigh muscles into your thighbones so that your legs become straight and strong but not tense. Ground the four corners of each foot – ball of the big toe, ball of the little toe, inner heel and outer heel – evenly and fully.**
- Lift the front of the pelvis upwards, keeping the spine vertical and the chest lifted. Keeping both feet firmly grounded, internally spiral the feet and legs, pressing back from the ball of the big toe along the inner edge of the foot to the inner heel, then the outer heel, in a rotating motion. Move the inner ankle bones back so that the groins move backwards, softening them and the buttocks. Move the inner edges of the knees outwards and broaden the pelvic floor.
- **Externally spiral the feet and legs, pressing out from the ball of the big toe to the ball of the little toe, and lengthening the outer edge of the foot, pressing back from the ball of the little toe to the outer heel. Move the outer knees backwards, drawing the outer hips back at the same time.**
- Engaging the bandhas, broaden and flatten your pubic abdomen, keeping your anus and core soft. Lengthen your abdomen, sucking your solar plexus in so that the ribcrests activate and broaden. Keep your abdominal muscles passive.
- **Keeping your weight even on your feet, and the left leg straight and spiralling from the foot, bend your right leg until you have a perfect right angle at the knee.**
- Keeping your right hand on your hip, extend your left arm forwards, rotating your spine and trunk, and place it on the right thigh by the knee.
- **Pressing with your left hand, make the pelvis and spine vertical. Roll your right shoulder back and look over it.**

Hold the posture – with feet, legs and bandhas maintaining the energetic and structural integrity of the posture; aware of the free flow of inhalation and exhalation; core soft – until ready to release. Repeat on the other side.

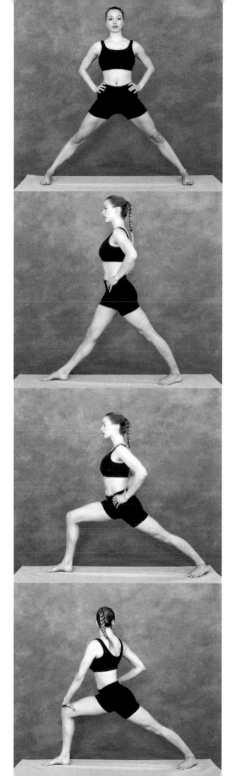

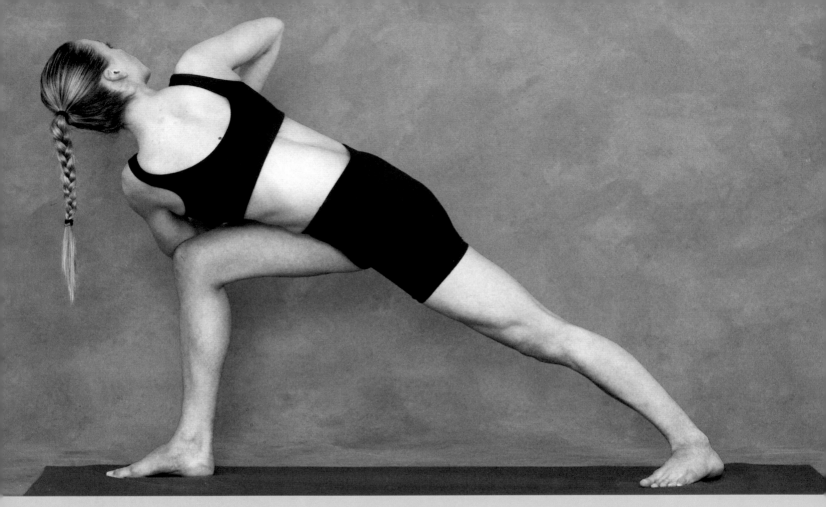

namaskarparsvakonasana

The feet are separated exactly so that when the front leg is bent you have a true right angle at the knee. The knee is directly above the heel, the thighbone is parallel to the floor, the shinbone perpendicular. The weight is even between the front and back foot, between the heels and the balls of the feet and between the inner and outer edges of the feet. The front buttock bone is kept tucked in by the right foot external spiral. The back leg is kept straight from the back foot internal spiral. The pelvis is kept in line from the back foot internal spiral. Place the bony point of the elbow against the outer bone of the front knee and use that contact, and that of the hands, to lift the trunk away from the leg and turn it. Keep the shoulders relaxed.

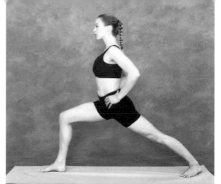

- Stand in hastatrikonasana with your hands on your hips.
- **Turn the right foot out exactly 90 degrees and the back foot in deeply enough to bring the back hip forward in line with the front hip. Suck the thigh muscles into your thighbones so that your legs become straight and strong but not tense. Ground the four corners of each foot – ball of the big toe, ball of the little toe, inner heel and outer heel – evenly and fully.**

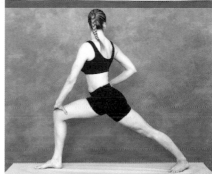

- Lift the front of the pelvis upwards, keeping the spine vertical and the chest lifted. Keeping both feet firmly grounded, internally spiral the feet and legs, pressing back from the ball of the big toe along the inner edge of the foot to the inner heel, then to the outer heel, in a rotating motion. Move the inner ankle bones back so that the groins move backwards, softening them and the buttocks. Move the inner edges of the knees outwards and broaden the pelvic floor.
- **Externally spiral the feet and legs, pressing out from the ball of the big toe to the ball of the little toe, and lengthening the outer edge of the foot, pressing back from the ball of the little toe to the outer heel. Move the outer knees backwards, drawing the outer hips back at the same time.**

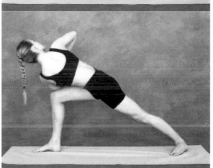

- Engaging the bandhas, broaden and flatten your pubic abdomen, keeping your anus and core soft. Lengthen your abdomen, sucking your solar plexus in so that the ribcrests activate and broaden. Keep your abdominal muscles passive.
- **Keeping your weight even on your feet, and the left leg straight and spiralling from the foot, bend your right leg until you have a perfect right angle at the knee.**
- Keeping your right hand on your hip, extend your left arm forwards, rotating your spine and trunk, and bring the armpit above the right knee.

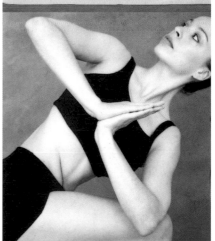

- **Bend your left arm and press the elbow point against the outer knee. Join the palms and extend the forearms in a vertical line.**
- From the internal spiral of your left foot, turn your right armpit towards the ceiling and look up along your right forearm.

Hold the posture – with feet, legs and bandhas maintaining the energetic and structural integrity of the posture; aware of the free flow of inhalation and exhalation; core soft – until ready to release. Repeat on the other side.

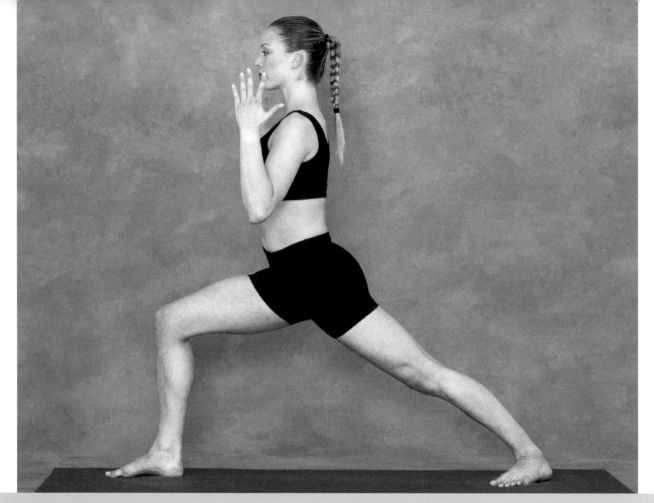

hastavirabadrasana

The feet are separated exactly so that when the front leg is bent you have a true right angle at the knee. The knee is directly above the heel, the thighbone is parallel to the floor, the shinbone perpendicular. The weight is even between the front and back foot, between the heels and the balls of the feet and between the inner and outer edges of the feet. The front buttock bone is kept tucked in by the right foot external spiral. The back leg is kept straight from the back foot internal spiral. The pelvis is kept in line from the back foot internal spiral. The pelvis is kept vertical from the grounding of the front foot. Use the arms to open the chest. Keep the shoulders relaxed, spine vertical.

- Stand in hastatrikonasana with your hands on your hips.
- **Turn the right foot out exactly 90 degrees and the back foot in deeply enough to bring the back hip forward in line with the front hip. Suck the thigh muscles into your thighbones so that your legs become straight and strong but not tense. Ground the four corners of each foot – ball of the big toe, ball of the little toe, inner heel and outer heel – evenly and fully.**
- Lift the front of the pelvis upwards, keeping the spine vertical and the chest lifted. Keeping both feet firmly grounded, internally spiral the feet and legs, pressing back from the ball of the big toe along the inner edge of the foot to the inner heel, then to the outer heel, in a rotating motion. Move the inner ankle bones back so that the groins move backwards, softening them and the buttocks. Move the inner edges of the knees outwards and broaden the pelvic floor.
- **Externally spiral the feet and legs, pressing out from the ball of the big toe to the ball of the little toe, and lengthening the outer edge of the foot, pressing back from the ball of the little toe to the outer heel. Move the outer knees backwards, drawing the outer hips back at the same time.**
- Engaging the bandhas, broaden and flatten your pubic abdomen, keeping your anus and core soft. Lengthen your abdomen, sucking your solar plexus in so that the ribcrests activate and broaden. Keep your abdominal muscles passive.
- **Keeping your weight even on your feet, and the left leg straight and spiralling from the foot, bend your right leg until you have a perfect right angle at the knee.**
- **Bend your arms, with your hands facing each other, fingers by the face, elbows tucked in by your ribs, and open your chest.**

Hold the posture – with feet, legs and bandhas maintaining the energetic and structural integrity of the posture; aware of the free flow of inhalation and exhalation; core soft – until ready to release. Repeat on the other side.

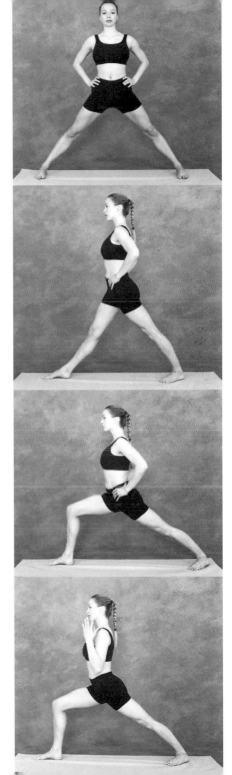

THE WARRIOR PRACTICE

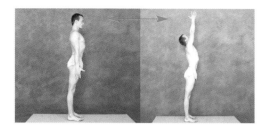

urdvahastulolla p108

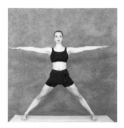

utktullola p108

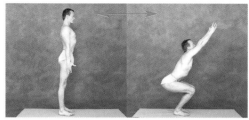

trikonasana p38

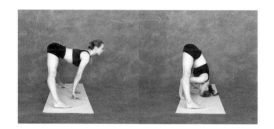

padottanullola p109

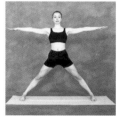

trikonasana p38

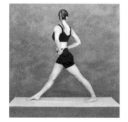

parivritasana p120

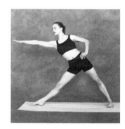

parsvasana p118

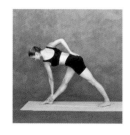

salambaparivritatrik-
onasana p124

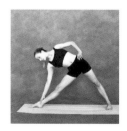

salambatrikon-
asana p122

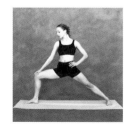

salambaparsvavira-
badrasana 134

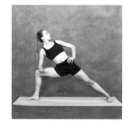

salambaparsvakon-
asana 136

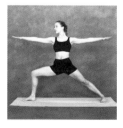

parsvavira-
badrasana p138

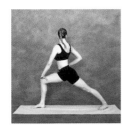 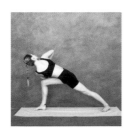 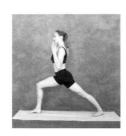 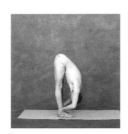 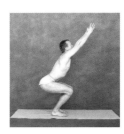

namaskarparsvak-
onasana p150

salambavirabadr-
asana p148

hastavirabadr-
asana p152

uttanasana p96

utktasana p96

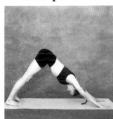 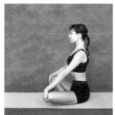 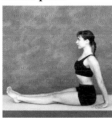 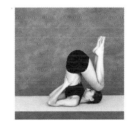 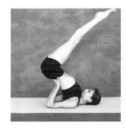

adomukasvan-
asana p82

dandasana p40

sukasana p24

ardapindasana p44

ardasarvangasana
asana p70

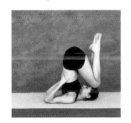 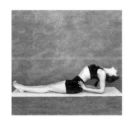 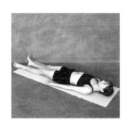 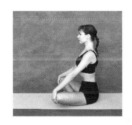

ardapindasana p44

ardamatsyasana p72

savasana p22

sukasana p24

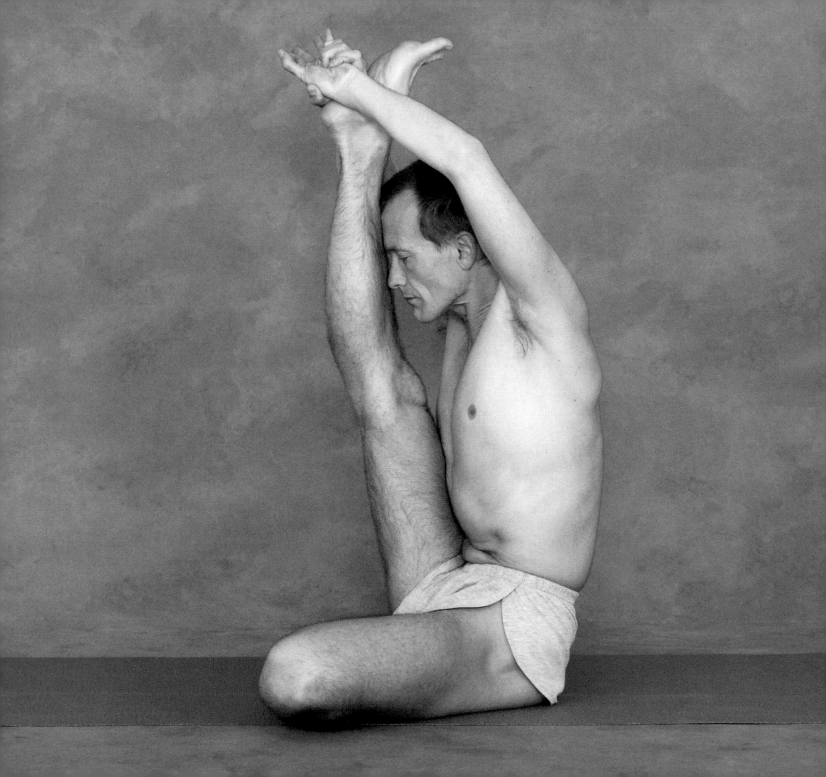

STRAIGHTENING THE LEGS

Hatha yoga postures can be divided into two broad categories. Those that open and restructure the body, compensating for misalignment, can be called the anatomical or restructuring postures. Those that open and nurture the body – cleansing, purifying, stimulating and balancing the organic and vital function – can be called the physiological or regenerating postures. However, the benefits of the second category are deeply enhanced by the work of the first. In fact, a yoga practice based primarily on the latter can easily create nervous instability and physical weakness. The first group is mainly represented by the standing postures, the second by those that are done with other parts of the body as the foundation. The first group releases more surface, anatomical tension; the second deeper, organic tension. The first group focuses more on the legs and pelvis, the second on the spine. Of course this distinction is only partly valid. It is more a differing emphasis than anything else, as all postures affect the anatomical and physiological functions of the body.

The three postures in this lesson are based on three standing postures, but are done from a sitting position. This allows them to be more easily held and more deeply penetrated, thus eliciting a deeper effect. Because of their structural impact, and the emphasis placed on the legs and pelvis rather than the spine, they can be used instead of standing postures to initiate a practice if you are tired. Because they are more easy to sustain than standing postures they offer a better opportunity to access and clarify the bandhas. This makes them more internalizing and opening than if they were done standing.

Even though the physical emphasis is on the raised leg, a strong emphasis can and should be given to the bandhas. These three postures clarify the dynamic relationship between the activity of the bandhas and their impact on the spine. They also clarify the dynamic interrelationship of the legs, pelvis and spine.

Isolating and activating only one leg, while keeping the spine centred and stable, allows an emphatic focus on the activity of the raised leg. This makes it possible to deeply penetrate the dynamic of leg and foot. This dynamic is, of course, no different to that of other postures. The shape of these postures, though, gives it a different quality; one which allows the practical dynamic of the legs and feet to be explored and clarified while in a non-strenuous posture. The leg is doing no supporting work that might trigger inappropriate, habitual muscular activity. The leg is right there in front of you. Exactly what you are doing is patently obvious.

The thigh muscles are sucked deeply into the bone so that the shin and thighbone line up. The ball of the foot is broadened, the inner and front ankle, the Achilles tendon and toes are extended. When the leg is engaged, it can then be used as a brace against which the arms can support the dynamic of the bandhas in lifting the chest and lengthening the waist. This is a triangular dynamic in which space is created between the three sides, as the trunk, spine and core lengthen from the activity of the bandhas, supported by the activity of the leg and the arms. The arms are actively lengthening spiralically, with the biceps rolling out and the base of the thumb gripping into the foot. The lift of the trunk is taken up the sides and into the armpits so they lift away from the hipbones, without disturbing the pelvis or lifting the shoulders. This is a universal action in the trunk that lengthens it and opens the chest. The armpits lift, the shoulders roll gently back and the shoulder blades go down the back. Tension should never be allowed into the shoulders.

urdvaikapadasana

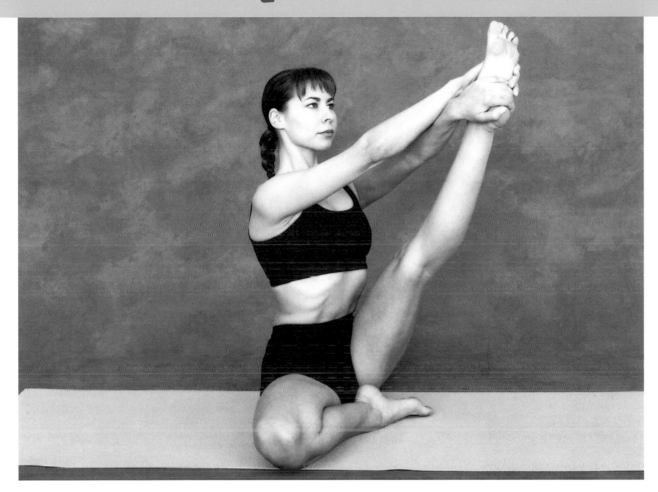

Raised-leg pose teaches the dynamic of a straight leg, and the relationship between the limbs and the trunk in the structural and energetic integrity emanating from the bandhas. It develops the legs and feet, releases the hamstrings and increases the mobility of the hip socket.

Raised-leg pose develops the feet and legs, opens the pelvis, releases the spine, relaxes the shoulders and opens the chest. Mulabandha stabilizes the lungs and sacrum, while uddiyanabandha lengthens the trunk, spine and core, opens the chest and protects the lower back. The spirallic action of the bandhas is transmitted clearly through the arms and raised leg, integrating the whole body effortlessly into a single energetic and structural dynamic.

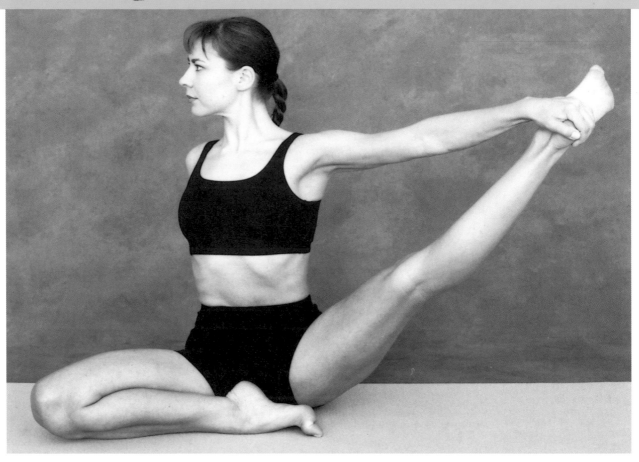

Side raised-leg pose teaches the dynamic of a straight leg, and the relationship between the limbs and the trunk in the structural and energetic integrity emanating from the bandhas. It develops the legs and feet, releases the hamstrings, inner thighs and groins and increases the mobility of the hip socket.

Side raised-leg pose develops the feet and legs, opens the pelvis, releases the spine, relaxes the shoulders and opens the chest. Mulabandha stabilizes the lungs and sacrum, while uddiyanabandha lengthens the trunk, spine and core, opens the chest and protects the lower back. The spirallic action of the bandhas is transmitted clearly through the arms and raised leg, integrating the whole body effortlessly into a single energetic and structural dynamic.

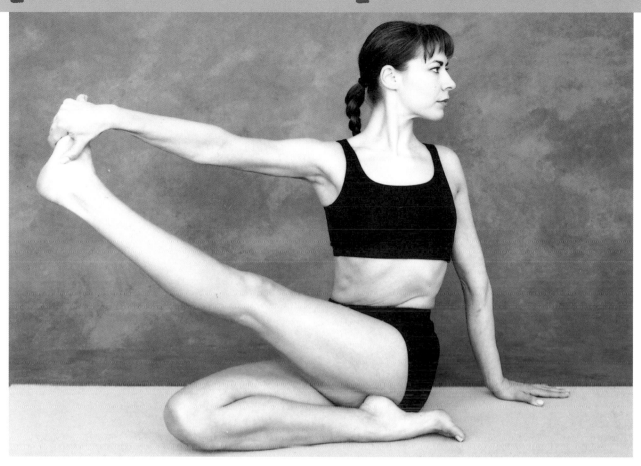

Twisting raised-leg pose teaches the dynamic of a straight leg, and the relationship between the limbs and the trunk in the structural and energetic integrity emanating from the bandhas. It develops the legs and feet, softens the back, releases the hamstrings and outer thighs and increases the mobility of the hip socket.

Twisting raised-leg pose develops the feet and legs, opens the pelvis, releases the spine, softens the back, mobilizes and nourishes the vertebrae, relaxes the shoulders and opens the chest. Mulabandha stabilizes the lungs and sacrum. Uddiyanabandha lengthens the trunk, spine and core, opens the chest and protects the lower back. The spirallic action of the bandhas is transmitted clearly through the arms and raised leg, integrating the whole body effortlessly into a single energetic and structural dynamic.

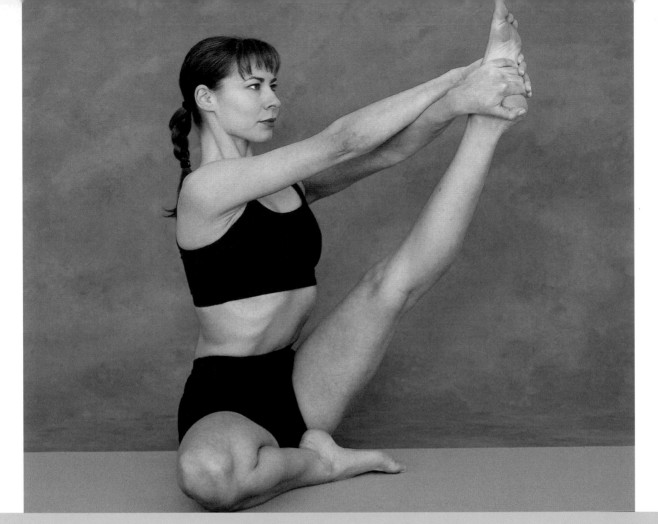

urdvaikapadasana

It is important for this posture that you sit on the front of the buttock bones. If you sit on the back of them you will not be able to engage the bandhas fully, lengthen the spine or open the chest. To try to do so from the back of the buttock bones will strain the lower back. The lower leg can be passive or the foot can be activated by broadening the ball of the foot and opening the ankle. The raised leg is active and straight, the foot alive. The bandhas are engaged; trunk, spine and core long; chest open; shoulders relaxed. Look at the raised foot.

- Sit with your legs crossed in sukasana.
- Draw your right heel into the pelvis.
- **Take the inner left heel in your left hand with the thumb down, and the outer left heel in your right hand with the thumb down so that your wrists are crossed over your front ankle.**
- Raise your left foot forwards and up in front of you.
- **Sucking your thigh muscles into the bone, straighten your leg and engage the foot by broadening the ball of the foot and lengthening through the front ankle, inner ankle, Achilles tendon and toes.** If you cannot straighten the leg, work with the leg bent until your hamstring lengthens, but keep using the thigh and the foot against the hands to try to straighten the leg as much as you can. This will maintain a lift into your trunk and spine.
- Broadening and flattening your pubic abdomen so the pelvic floor is passively lifted, engage mulabandha. Broaden the ribcrests, suck the solar plexus in with the abdomen passive, and engage uddiyanabandha. Come to the front edge of your buttock bones.
- **Clarify the action of the left leg, thighs sucked in, foot alive**.
- Rolling your shoulders back, lengthen and spiral your arms, lift your armpits and relax your shoulders. Look at your foot.

Hold the posture – with your left leg and foot engaged; aware of the free flow of inhalation and exhalation; abdomen passive, long and hollow; solar plexus sucked in; chest broad and active; pubic abdomen flat and broad; anus and core soft – until ready to release. Repeat on the other side.

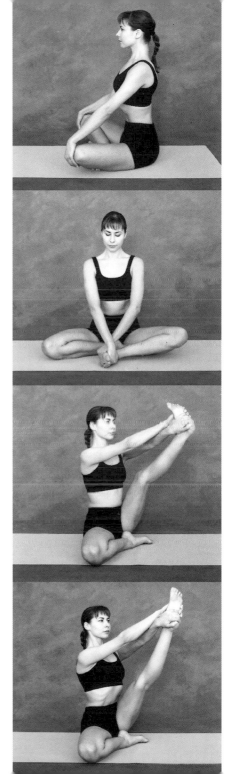

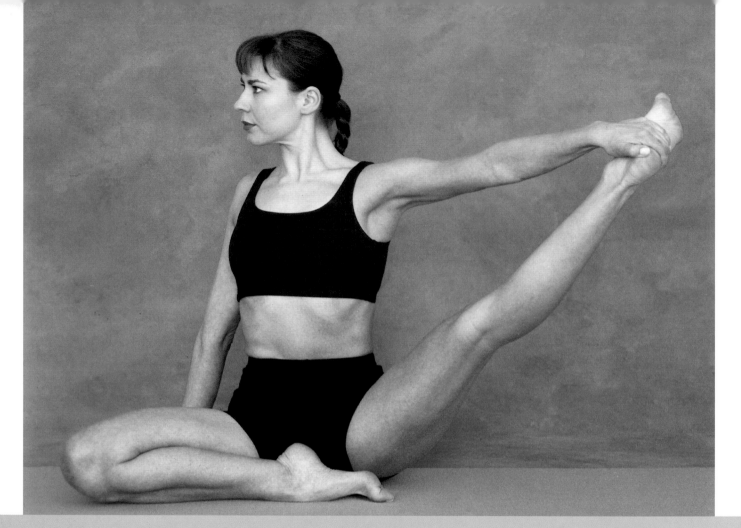

parsvaikapadasana

It is important for this posture that you sit on the front of the buttock bones. If you sit on the back of them you will not be able to engage the bandhas fully, lengthen the spine or open the chest. To try to do so from the back of the buttock bones will strain the lower back. The lower leg can be passive or the foot can be activated by broadening the ball of the foot and opening the ankle. The raised leg is active and straight, the foot alive. The bandhas are engaged; trunk, spine and core long; chest open; shoulders relaxed. Look at the raised foot.

- Sit with your legs crossed in sukasana.
- Draw your right heel into the pelvis.
- **Take the inner left heel in your left hand with the thumb down and place your right hand on the floor by your right buttock.**
- Raise your left foot forwards and up in front of you.
- **Sucking your thigh muscles into the bone, straighten your leg and engage the foot by broadening the ball of the foot and lengthening through the front ankle, inner ankle, Achilles tendon and toes.** If you cannot straighten the leg, work with the leg bent until your hamstring lengthens, but keep using the thigh and the foot against the hand to try to straighten the leg as much as you can. This will maintain a lift into your trunk and spine.
- Broadening and flattening your pubic abdomen so the pelvic floor is passively lifted, engage mulabandha. Broaden the ribcrests, suck the solar plexus in with the abdomen passive, and engage uddiyanabandha. Come to the front edge of your buttock bones.
- **Rolling your shoulders back, lengthen and spiral your arms, lift your armpits and relax your shoulders.**
- Place your right hand on the floor by your right buttock and, keeping leg and foot engaged and both buttock bones on the floor, take your leg out to the left as far as possible. Resist the tendency of the foot to roll outwards as much as you can.
- **Turn your head slowly to the right as you use the triangular dynamic to lengthen the trunk, spine and core.**

Hold the posture – with your left leg and foot engaged; aware of the free flow of inhalation and exhalation; abdomen passive, long and hollow; solar plexus sucked in; chest broad and active; pubic abdomen flat and broad; anus and core soft – until ready to release. Repeat on the other side.

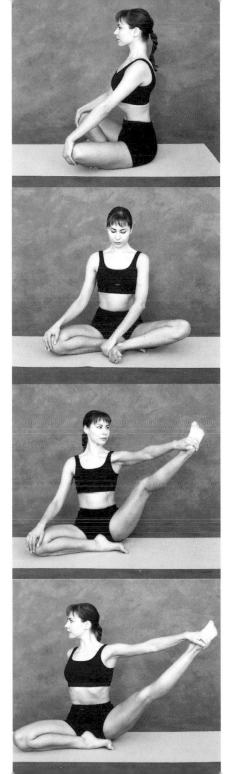

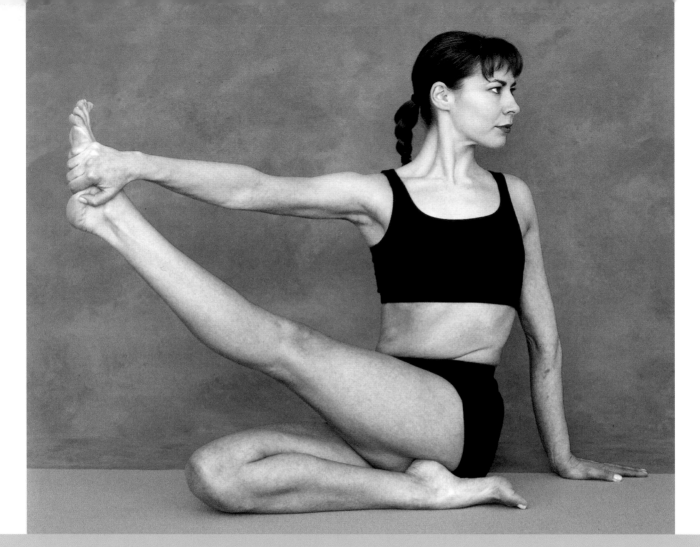

parivritaikapadasana

It is important for this posture that you sit on the front of the buttock bones. If you sit on the back of them you will not be able to engage the bandhas fully, lengthen the spine or open the chest. To try to do so from the back of the buttock bones will strain the lower back. The lower leg can be passive or the foot can be activated by broadening the ball of the foot and opening the ankle. The raised leg is active and straight, the foot alive. The bandhas are engaged; trunk, spine and core long; chest open; shoulders relaxed.

- Sit with your legs crossed in sukasana.
- Draw your right heel into the pelvis.
- **Take the outer left heel in your right hand with the thumb down and place your left hand on the floor by your left buttock.**
- Raise your left foot forwards and up in front of you.
- **Sucking your thigh muscles into the bone, straighten your leg and engage the foot by broadening the ball of the foot and lengthening through the front ankle, inner ankle, Achilles tendon and toes.** If you cannot straighten the leg, work with the leg bent until your hamstring lengthens, but keep using the thigh and the foot against the hand to try to straighten the leg as much as you can. This will maintain a lift into your trunk and spine.
- Broadening and flattening your pubic abdomen so the pelvic floor is passively lifted, engage mulabandha. Broaden the ribcrests, suck the solar plexus in with the abdomen passive, and engage uddiyanabandha. Come to the front edge of your buttock bones.
- **Rolling your shoulders back, lengthen and spiral your arms, lift your armpits and relax your shoulders.**
- Keeping leg and foot engaged and both buttock bones on the floor, take the foot to the right, across the line of your body.
- **Turn your head slowly to the left as you use the triangular dynamic to lengthen the trunk, spine and core.**

Hold the posture – with your left leg and foot engaged; aware of the free flow of inhalation and exhalation; abdomen passive, long and hollow; solar plexus sucked in; chest broad and active; pubic abdomen flat and broad; anus and core soft – until ready to release. Repeat on the other side.

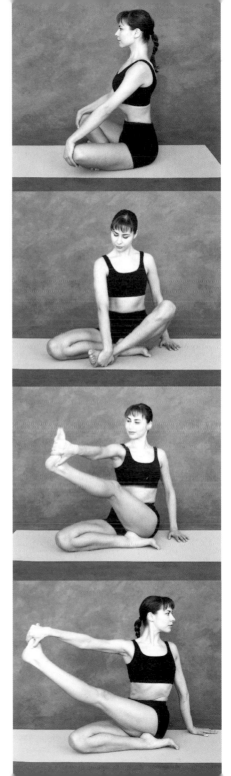

THE RAISED LEG PRACTICE

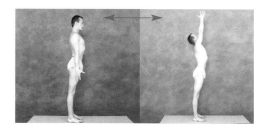
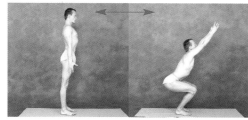
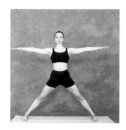

urdvahastullola p108   utktullola p108   trikonasana p38

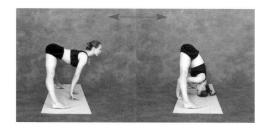
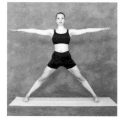
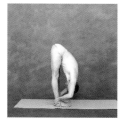
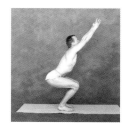

padottanullola p109   trikonasana p38   uttanasana p96   utktasana p96

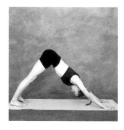
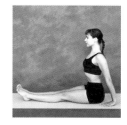
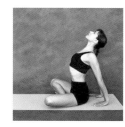
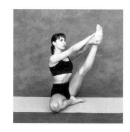
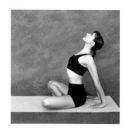

adomukasvan-   dandasana p40   chakrasukasana   urdvaikapad-   chakrasukasana
asana p82   p25   asana p160   p25

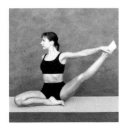

parsvaikapad-
asana p164

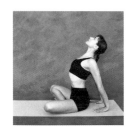

chakrasukasana
p25

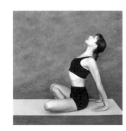

parivritaikapad-
asana p166

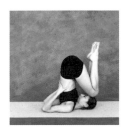

chakrasukasana
p25

ardapindasana p44

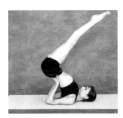

ardasarvang-
asana p70

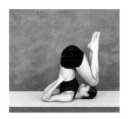

ardapindasana p44

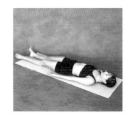

ardamatsyasana p72

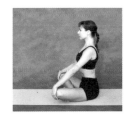

savasana p22

sukasana p24

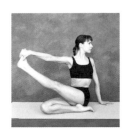

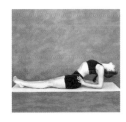

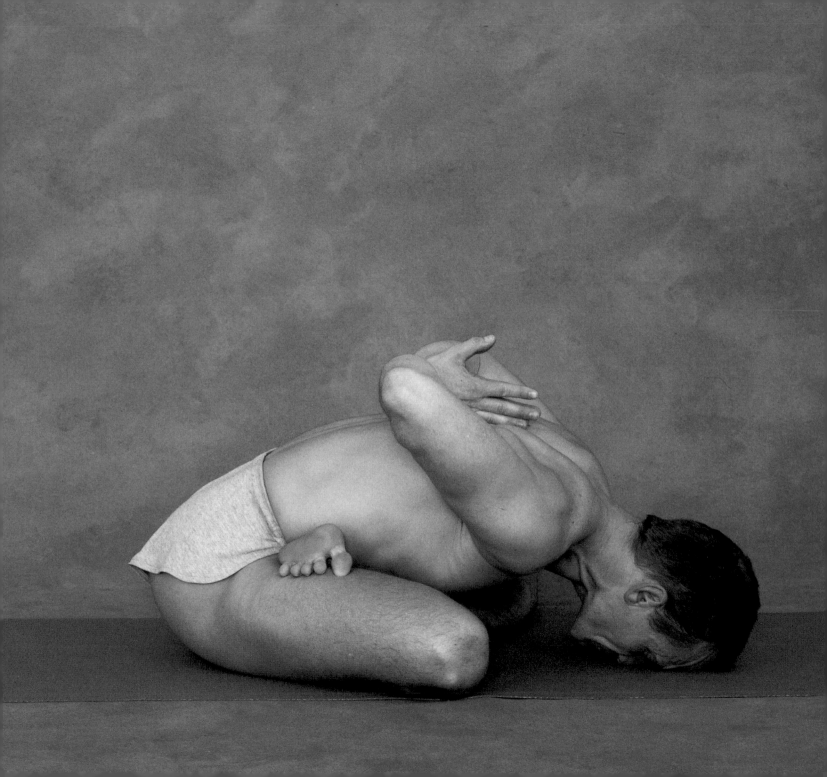

RELEASING THE SPINE

The spine is the anatomical key of hatha yoga. The vertical extension of the spine is completely natural and inherently requires no effort. Unfortunately, few of us are able to experience this. Tension in the trunk pulls this way and that on the spine, restricting its ability to extend. Once our body is free from tension, however, the spine assumes its natural tendency to elevate upwards. Yoga, by freeing the spine's supporting muscles of all tension, reawakens this natural capacity of the spine to extend effortlessly.

We begin this lesson with two vertical extensions. In their classical form they are forward extensions also, but the positions of the legs make them far more challenging than many other forward extensions. The next two postures are forward extensions. It is absolutely NOT important how close you bring your chest to your legs or your head to your feet. What is important is that you activate the spirallic adjustments of each part of the body to express the dynamic of the bandhas as fully and evenly as you can. All four of these postures must be grounded on the front edge of the buttock bones. This is to allow the posture to originate in the pelvis, not the back. The last posture also extends the trunk and spine, but more obviously.

Remember to keep your foundation grounded throughout. With the exception of the second posture, the legs and feet remain spirally engaged. At the same time, of course, remember to keep the core soft and the bandhas engaged, while resonating their dynamic throughout your whole body. Keep your shoulders relaxed as your armpits lift and spine lengthens.

urdvakonasana

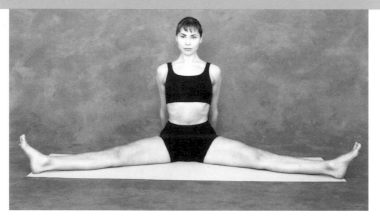

Sitting splits teaches the dynamic use of the legs as a foundation for extending the spine. It therefore teaches the importance of the foundation in releasing the spine and opening the chest. It also teaches the spirallic use of the arms to support the elevation of the trunk, spine and core, thus facilitating breathing.

Sitting splits develops the legs and feet, lengthens the hamstrings, opens the groins and stimulates circulation to the pelvis and the reproductive organs. Mulabandha stabilizes the lungs and sacrum, while uddiyanabandha lengthens the trunk, spine and core, opens the chest and protects the lower back.

urdvabadakonasana

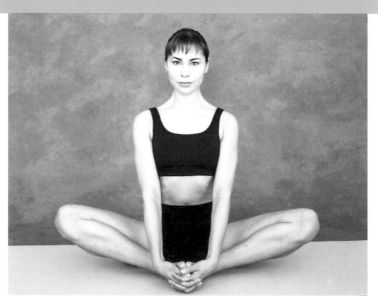

Sitting cobbler teaches the dynamic use of the arms as supports to the bandhas for extending the spine. It therefore teaches the importance of the foundation in releasing the spine and opening the chest. It also teaches the spirallic use of the arms to support the elevation of the trunk, spine and core, thus facilitating breathing.

It lengthens the inner thighs, and opens the groins and hips. It stimulates circulation to the pelvis and reproductive organs. Mulabandha stabilizes the lungs and sacrum, while uddiyan-abandha lengthens the trunk, spine and core, opens the chest and protects the lower back.

pascimasana

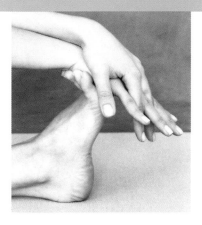 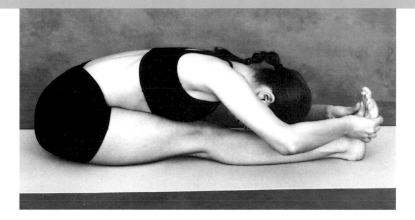

One-leg-forward extension teaches how to initiate a forward extension from the pelvis and use the band-has to extend the front of the body, while closing it. It mobilizes the pelvis, lengthens the hamstrings, opens the hips and releases the spine and back. It internalizes energy and attention, soothes the nerves, quiets the mind and challenges emotional blocks. Mulabandha stabilizes the lungs and sacrum, while uddiyanabandha lengthens the trunk, spine and core, opens the chest and protects the lower back.

The best hand grip to use, when possible, is to place the centre of the right palm over the ball of the foot with the fingers spread. The left hand is then placed on top, with its fingers in the spaces between the fingers of the right hand. Keep both hands open and dynamically expressing the bandhas, as you use the hand-foot contact to extend the spine forwards. This may not be possible to begin with.

pascimottanasana

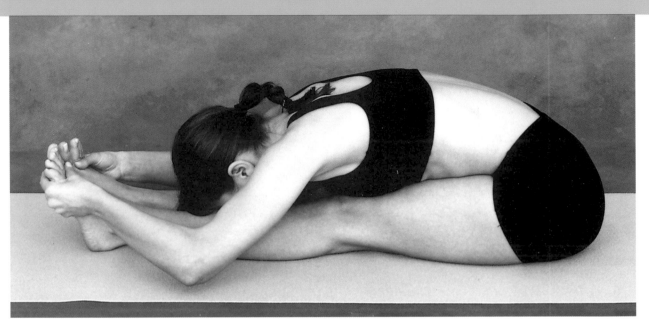

Forward extension teaches how to initiate a forward extension from the pelvis and how to use the bandhas to extend the front of the body while closing it. It mobilizes the pelvis, lengthens the hamstrings and releases the spine and back. It internalizes energy and attention, soothes the nerves, quiets the mind and challenges emotional blocks.

Mulabandha stabilizes the lungs and sacrum, while uddiyanabandha lengthens the trunk, spine and core, opens the chest and protects the lower back.

purvottanasana

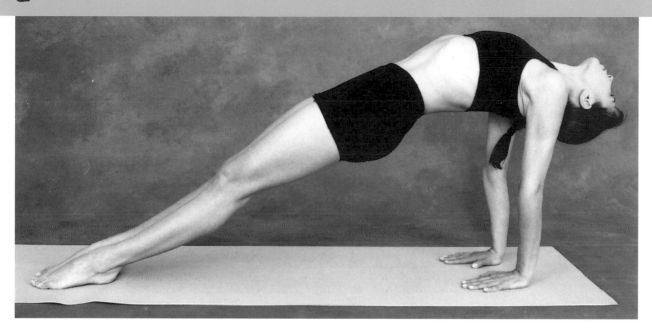

Opening pose teaches how to lengthen the fronts of the legs and how to spiral the arm to support and open the chest. It lengthens the front thighs, groins and waist; mobilizes the ankles; stretches the arch of the feet; develops the hands, wrists and arms; engages the thoracic spine and opens the chest. It energizes the nerves, sharpens the mind and opens the heart.

Mulabandha stabilizes the lungs and sacrum, while uddiyanabandha lengthens the trunk, spine and core, opens the chest and protects the lower back.

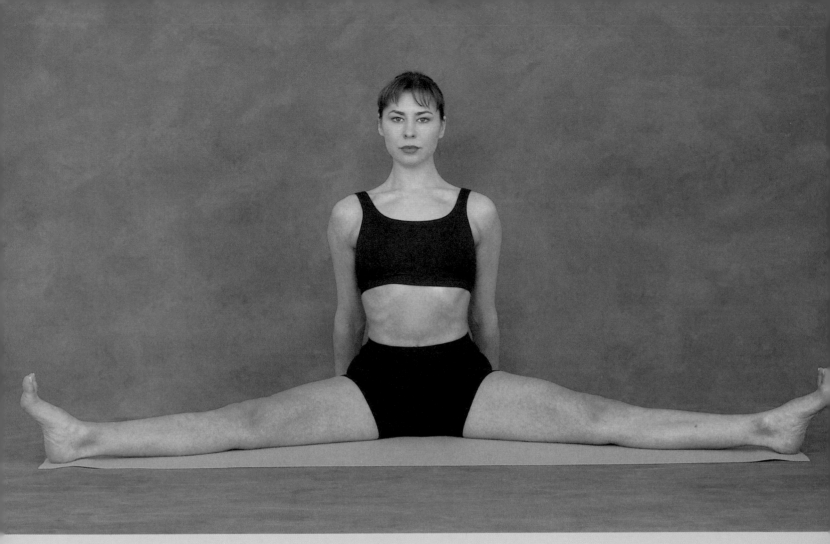

urdvakonasana

With your legs dynamically engaged, spiral them from the feet so that both the inner and outer knees go down and the thighs remain centred. Keep the feet on the centre of the heels. On the front edges of your buttockbones use the hands and arms to support the lengthening effect of the bandhas on the trunk, spine and core. Keep your shoulders relaxed as you lengthen your waist, taking your armpits away from your hipbones.

- Sit with your legs relaxed in front of you.
- **Taking your feet as far from each other as possible, spread your legs wide apart.**
- Placing your hands behind your buttocks, lift your buttocks off the floor and, pushing your groins forward, spread your legs even wider.
- **Pressing your palms into the floor behind your buttocks, engage the feet and thighs, pressing the legs down into the floor with the feet centred on the heels.**
- Use the hands to bring you to the front edge of your buttock bones. Broadening and flattening your pubic abdomen, so the pelvic floor is passively lifted, engage mulabandha. Broadening the ribcrests, suck the solar plexus in, with the abdomen passive, and engage uddiyanabandha.
- **Pressing with the bases of your index fingers, spiral the arms and lengthen the waist, taking your armpits away from your ears as you relax your shoulders.**
- Look straight ahead.

Hold the posture – with your feet and legs engaged; aware of the free flow of inhalation and exhalation; abdomen passive, long and hollow; solar plexus sucked in, chest broad and active; pubic abdomen flat and broad; anus and core soft – until ready to release.

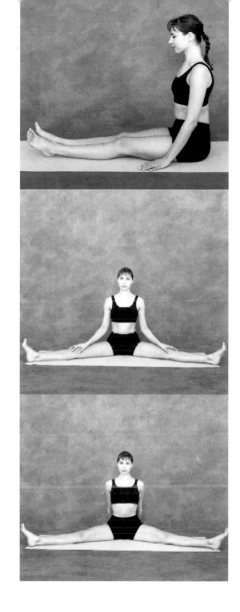

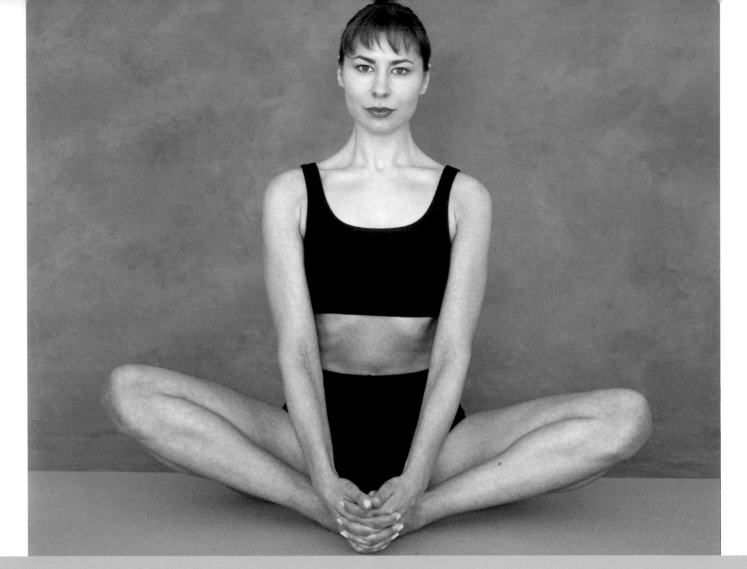

urdvabadakonasana

The legs are relaxed, with the feet pressing together firmly but without aggression. The hands and arms support the lift of the trunk. Sit on the front edge of the buttock bones and create a strong dynamic between the arms, feet and trunk, keeping your shoulders relaxed and your spine lengthened.

- Sit with your legs crossed in front of you.
- **Take hold of each foot with your hands.**
- Bringing the soles of your feet together, join the balls of your feet and your heels.
- **Interlock your fingers and wrap them around the balls of your feet and your toes, and press the feet together.**
- Come to the front edge of your buttock bones and, broadening and flattening your pubic abdomen so the pelvic floor is passively lifted, engage mulabandha. Broadening the ribcrests, suck the solar plexus in, with the abdomen passive, and engage uddiyanabandha.
- **Press your feet together, spiral your arms, roll your shoulders back and lengthen you waist.**
- Look straight ahead.

Hold the posture – arms engaged; aware of the free flow of inhalation and exhalation; core soft; abdomen passive, long and hollow; solar plexus sucked in; chest broad and active; pubic abdomen flat and broad; anus soft – until ready to release.

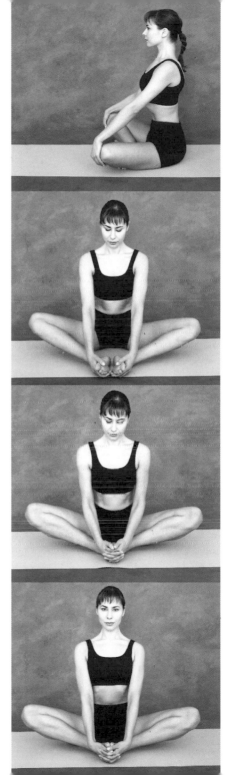

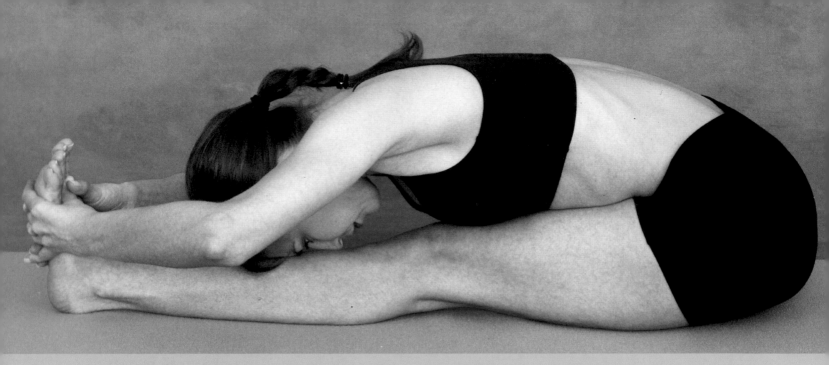

pascimasana

Great care must be taken when bending the passive leg and positioning its foot. Knees are very vulnerable joints and can easily be irritated to the point of injury by consistently insensitive practice. When extending the spine forward parallel to the floor, the passive leg is potentially at risk. To protect the connective tissue of the knee, the joint must be tightly closed. This allows the leg to relax and protects the connective tissues. If the knee joint is not fully closed because the foot cannot be drawn far enough back, or the shinbone is not tight into the thighbone, then the forward movement brings weight onto the unsupported knee joint, putting pressure on its connective tissue. This causes incremental irritation that can lead, without warning, to serious injury. The method given here for bending the passive leg should be used in all other one-leg-forward extensions in which the passive leg is placed in a similar manner. It should also be used for both legs entering full lotus, and for half lotus posture and its variations. When drawing the bent leg groin in towards the straight leg groin, make sure that the shinbone does not rotate up and in towards you, pinching in the front corner of the knee. In some cases this requires resistance on the shinbone from the hands. The right heel is placed in the left groin, foot against the thigh, not under it – do not force yourself forwards or down, you will strain your lower back. Be patient and learn how to use the foundation and the bandhas to challenge your limitations and increase your capability without aggression. The lower back should not flatten and harden. The whole spine should be gently rounded so that the back can relax. Relax the neck so that the weight of your head can pull on and lengthen your back muscles.

- Sit on the floor with your legs relaxed in front of you.
- **Keeping the legs relaxed, take hold of the back of your right knee with your right hand and your right foot with your left hand.**
- Leaning away from your left leg, slip your right hand down the right shin, draw the right shin tight into the right thighbone, and let your right knee come to the floor. If the knee cannot come to the floor with the leg completely relaxed, place a block, book or blankets under it for support so the leg can completely relax.
- **Place your right heel in the left groin, with the foot running along the inner edge of the left thigh.**
- Take your hands behind your buttocks and bring yourself to the front edge of the buttock bones.
- **Facing your left foot, engage and straighten the left leg by sucking the thigh muscles into the bone. Broaden the ball of the foot and open the ankle, pressing the knees and heels to the floor.**
- Broadening and flattening your pubic abdomen so the pelvic floor is passively lifted, engage mulabandha. Broadening the ribcrests, suck the solar plexus in, with the abdomen passive, and engage uddiyanabandha.
- **Pivot your pelvis forwards so the pubic bone and buttock bones roll back as the hipbones roll forward. Reach forwards as far as you can, lengthening your arms without bending your leg, and catch hold of the shinbone, ankle, sides of the feet or ball of the foot.**
- Keeping your leg straight, lift your head from the chin, roll the shoulders back and extend the armpits forwards and up. Roll the pubic bone back and lengthen the front of your body as you clarify the bandhas.
- **Allow the trunk to keep its length as you continue to take the pubic bone back and extend your trunk along the line of the leg, dropping your head towards your leg.**

Hold the posture – with your leg and foot engaged; aware of the free flow of inhalation and exhalation; core soft; abdomen passive, long and hollow; solar plexus sucked in; chest broad and active; pubic abdomen flat and broad; anus soft – until ready to release. Repeat on the other side.

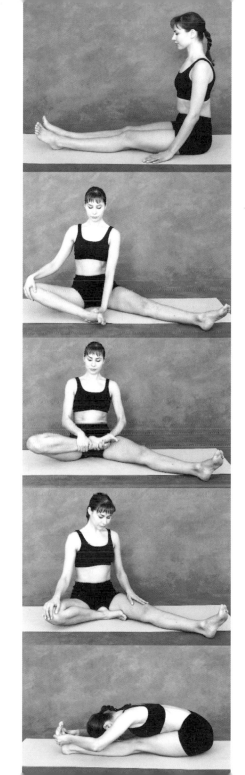

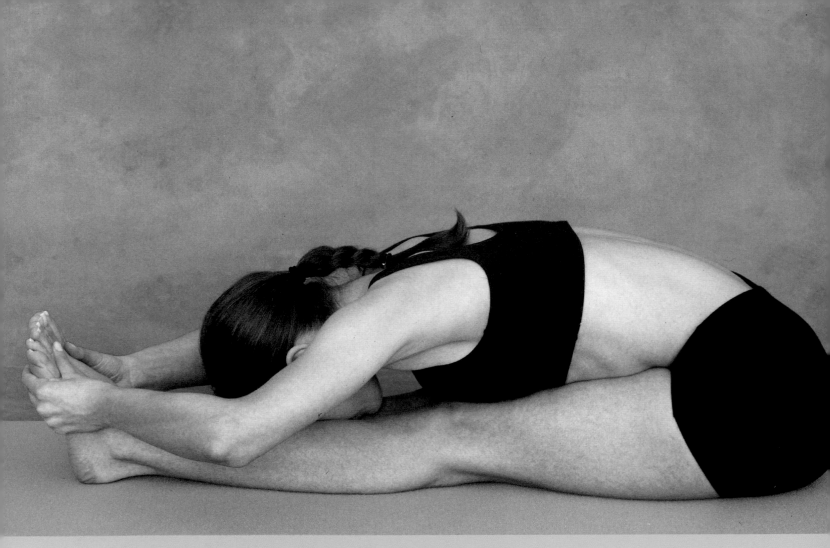

pascimottanasana

Do not force yourself forwards or down, as this will strain your lower back. Be patient and learn how to use the foundation and the bandhas to challenge your limitations and increase your capability without aggression. The lower back should not flatten and harden. The whole spine should be gently rounded so that the back can relax. Relax the neck so that the weight of your head can pull on and lengthen your back muscles.

- Sit on the floor with your legs relaxed in front of you.
- Take your hands behind your buttocks, and bring yourself to the front edge of the buttock bones.
- **Facing your feet, engage and straighten the legs, grounding your heels and knees by sucking the thigh muscles into the bone. Broaden the balls of the feet, open the ankles and press the backs of the heels down.**
- Broadening and flattening your pubic abdomen so the pelvic floor is passively lifted, engage mulabandha. Broadening the ribcrests, suck the solar plexus in, with the abdomen passive, and engage uddiyanabandha.
- **Pivot your pelvis forwards so the pubic bone and buttock bones roll back as the hipbones roll forward. Reach forwards as far as you can, lengthening your arms without bending your legs, and catch hold of the shinbone, ankle, sides of the feet or ball of the foot.**
- Keeping your legs straight, lift your head from the chin, roll the shoulders back and extend the armpits forwards and up. Roll the pubic bone back and lengthen the front of your body as you clarify the bandhas.
- **Allow the trunk to keep its length as you continue to take the pubic bone back and extend your trunk along the line of the legs, dropping your head down towards your legs.**

Hold the posture – with your legs and feet engaged; aware of the free flow of inhalation and exhalation; abdomen passive, long and hollow; solar plexus sucked in, chest broad and active; pubic abdomen flat and broad; core and anus soft – until ready to release.

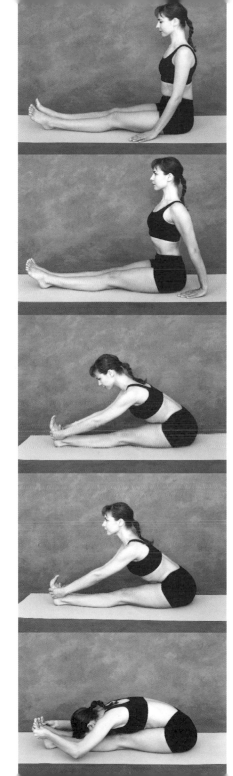

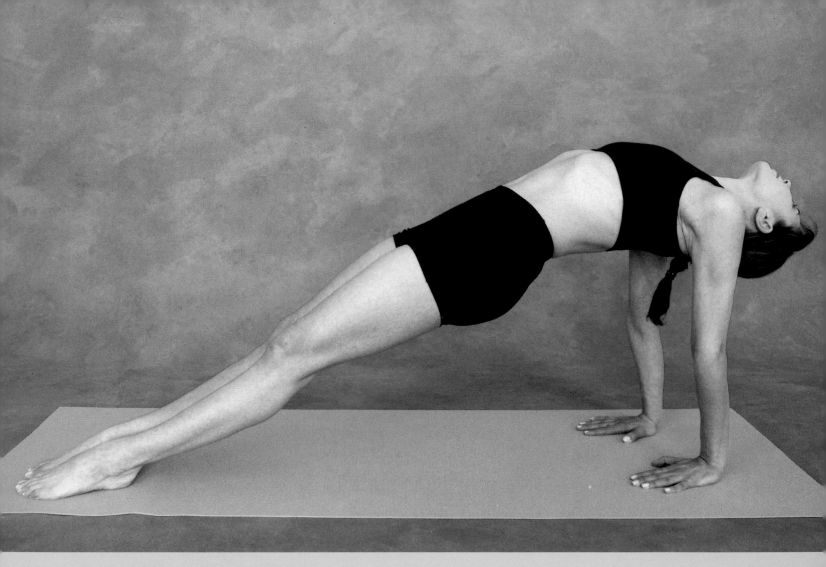

purvottanasana

Keep the front of the body fully extended, spiralling your arms from your hands to lift and hold you. Keep the bandhas engaged, top spine lifting into the chest. Try to bring the inner edges of the feet together and the balls of the feet onto the floor.

- Sit in dandasana.
- **Suck the thigh muscles into the thighbones so that the kneecaps are pulled up and in, the knee bones go down and the shin and thigh bones line up. Engage the feet.**
- Place your hands behind your buttocks so the fingers point towards the feet.
- **Press down into the floor with the bases of your fingers and the heels of your hands. Roll your shoulders back and lift your top spine forwards into the chest.**
- Broadening and flattening your pubic abdomen so the pelvic floor is passively lifted, engage mulabandha. Broadening the ribcrests, suck the solar plexus in, with the abdomen passive, and engage uddiyanabandha.
- **Keeping your legs strong, press with your hands and raise the buttocks as high as you can, keeping the dynamic in the trunk.**
- Lift your head up from the base of the skull, rotating the chin forwards, up and then back.

Hold the posture – with your legs and arms engaged; aware of the free flow of inhalation and exhalation; abdomen passive, long and hollow; solar plexus sucked in; chest broad and active; pubic abdomen flat and broad; anus soft – until ready to release.

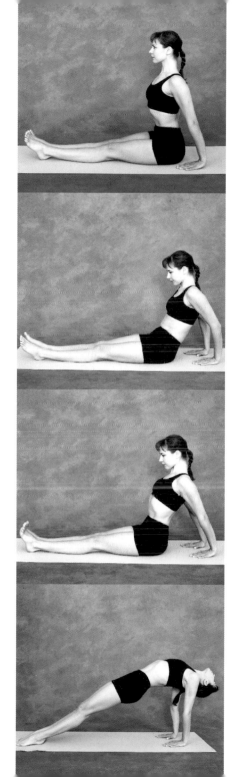

THE EXTENSION PRACTICE

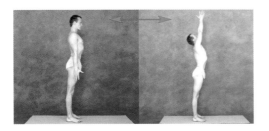

urdvahastullola p108

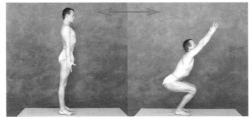

utktullola p108

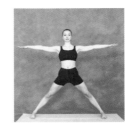

trikonasana p38

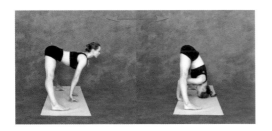

padottanullola p109

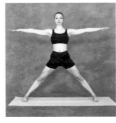

trikonasana p38

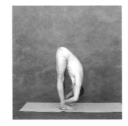

uttanasana p96

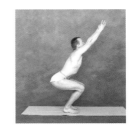

utktasana p96

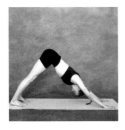

adomukasvan-
asana p82

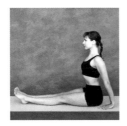

dandasana p40

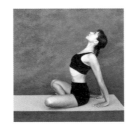

chakrasukasana p25

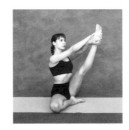

urdvaikapadasana
p162

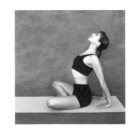

chakrasukasana p25

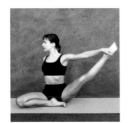

parsvaikapadasana
p164

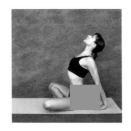

chakrasukasana p25

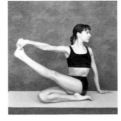

parivritaikapad-
asana p166

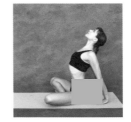

chakrasukasana p25

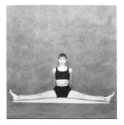

urdvakonasana p176

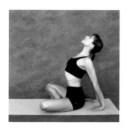 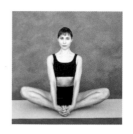 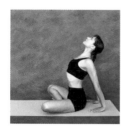 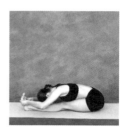 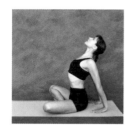

chakrasukasana p25 urdvabadakon- chakrasukasana p25 pascimasana p180 chakrasukasana 25
asana p178

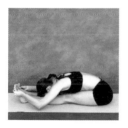 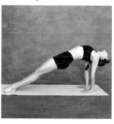 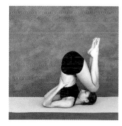 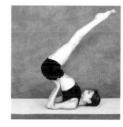 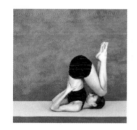

pascimottanasana purvottanasana ardapindasana p44 ardasarvangasana ardapindasana p44
p182 p184 p70

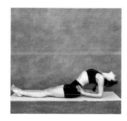 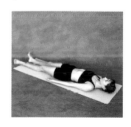 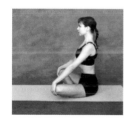

ardamatsyasana p72 savasana p22 sukasana p24

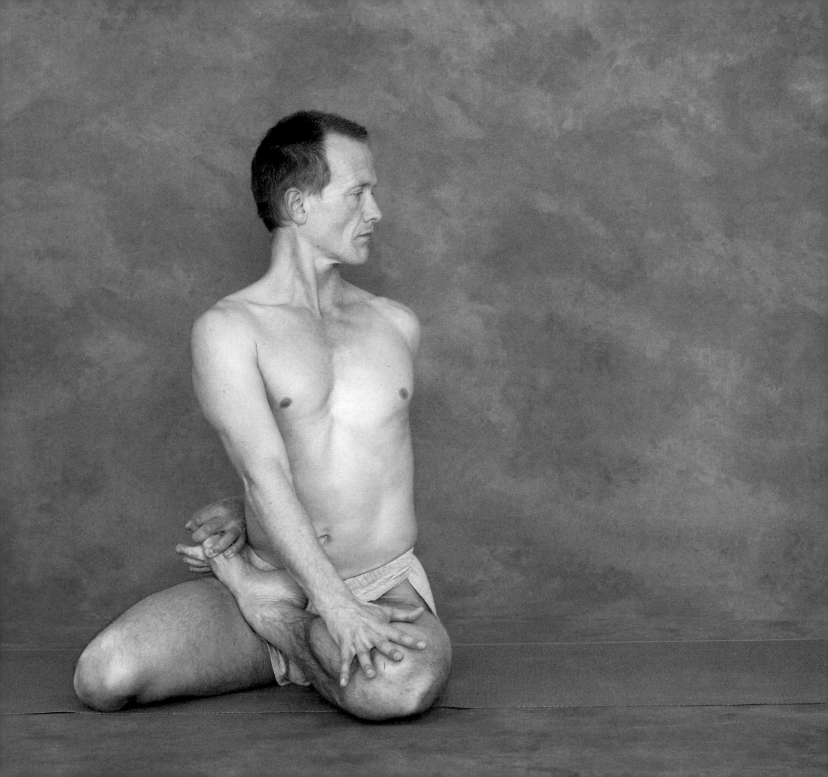

SOFTENING THE BACK

Rotations of the spine are vital. They mobilize the intervertebral spaces, increasing blood supply to the spinal cord. This is especially vital to people of 35 years and older, whose spinal blood supply is becoming restricted as the intervertebral spaces close and seize up. Spinal rotations and twists, by maintaining intervertebral mobility, slow this process down and delay ageing. They also keep the back muscles soft. This makes rotations beneficial as counterposes, and as preparations for the intense extensions and flexions of forward bends and backbends. Unfortunately, these more extreme movements very often result in tightening of muscles, either as a result of poor physical technique, or exacerbation of existing but overlooked problems. Rotations and twists then become even more necessary to a balanced yoga practice.

Rotations and twists are not so much about establishing movement, as maintaining it. Pushing for extra movement in twists is especially inappropriate, as their purpose is to soften, rest and recharge the muscles. They are physically gentle postures. Internally, however, they can be very intense. They can create a lot of heat, as well as instantaneous shifts in awareness and internalization. Because seated twists are also very stable, they invite extended stillness. This, in turn, promotes deep internalization and inner quietness. They are a great place to learn attentiveness and sensitivity, and to focus on stillness, the bandhas and the breath.

The first two postures in this lesson are rotations rather than twists, the third is a twist. The difference between the two is that in a rotation the whole spine moves in the same direction, whereas in a twist the top spine moves one way, the bottom the other. Twists offer much greater movement than rotations. They are also therefore potentially more of a risk. On the other hand, the fact that the lower back will not rotate as freely as the neck and the upper back means that rotations can easily degenerate into twists if ambition overcomes attentiveness. When doing any rotations be sure to move slowly, initiating the rotation from the lower spine while keeping the foundation stable. As you rotate, pay attention to the navel. If you begin to feel that the skin above the navel is separating from the skin below the navel, as the upper spine begins to access a movement not available to the lower spine, release a little until this sensation is no longer present. In the last posture, enjoy the greater movement available in a twist but be sensitive to your lower and middle back. In all cases, do not force your body to go further. Twists are great places to learn how to use duration and the breath to find and extend the body's capacity. By working more on extending the spine, rather than turning it, and staying with the flow of your breathing, you will access whatever movement is currently available. You can then let go of any preconceived ideas about how far you should or could move, and surrender to the actuality of your current capability.

sukamaricyasana

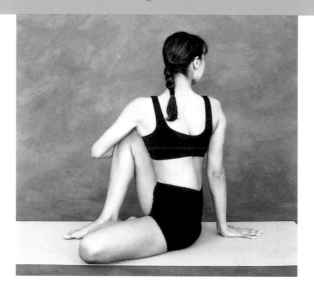

Easy rotation teaches the art of extending in order to rotate and the art of extending the spine in order to breathe more freely. It also teaches the spirallic use of the hand and arm in opening the chest and facilitating breathing.

Easy rotation frees the pelvis, softens the back and spine, mobilizes the neck vertebrae and challenges the breath. Mulabandha stabilizes the lungs and the sacrum, while uddiyanabandha protects the lower back, lengthens the spine and core and opens the chest.

maricyasana

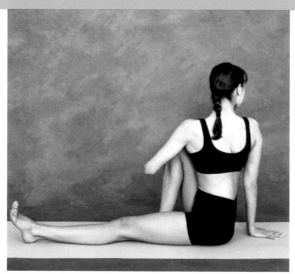

Seated rotation teaches the art of extending in order to rotate and the art of extending the spine in order to breathe more freely. It teaches the power of the foundation to support extension, and thereby rotation. It also teaches the spirallic use of the hand and arm in opening the chest and facilitating breathing.

Seated rotation frees the pelvis, softens the back and spine, mobilizes the neck vertebrae and challenges the breath. Mulabandha stabilizes the lungs and the sacrum, while uddiyanabandha protects the lower back, lengthens the spine and core and opens the chest.

suptaparivritasana

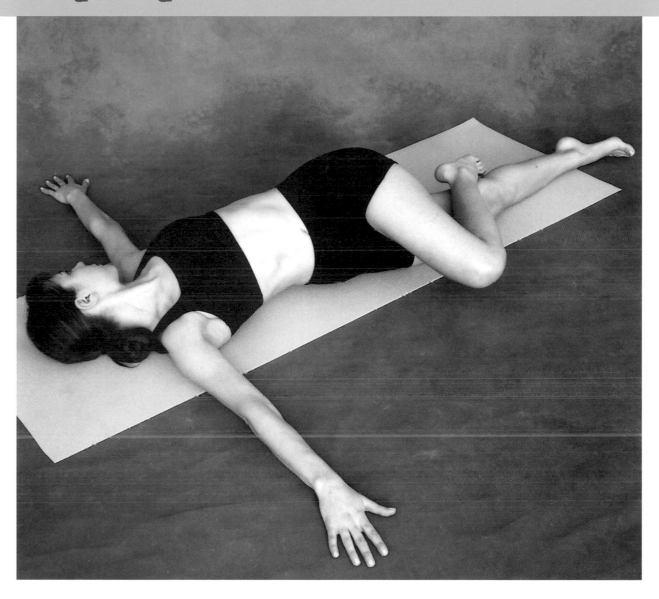

Lying twist teaches the art of letting go in order to soften and twist. It relaxes the whole body, softens the back and spine, mobilizes the neck and challenges the breath.

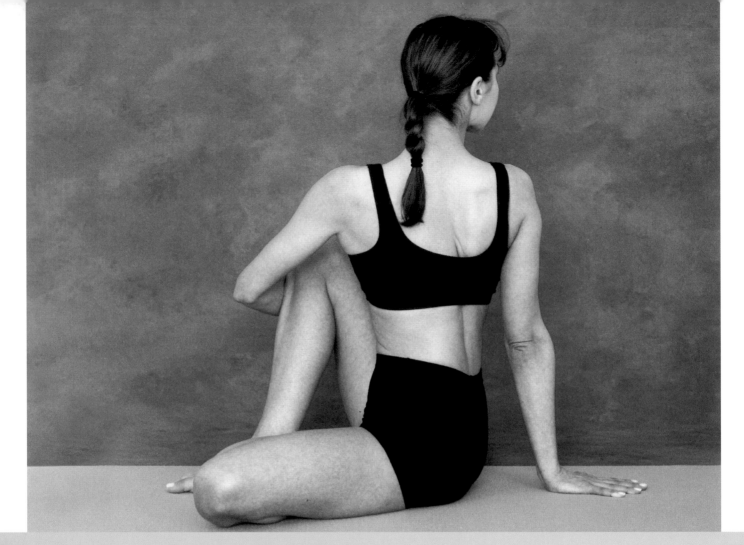

sukamaricyasana

The bottom leg is allowed to become completely passive, while the foot of the top leg presses into the floor as an active part of the foundation. The front of the buttock bones and the leading hand and arm are also part of the dynamic of the foundation. The hand of the 'wrapping' arm is kept alive and open. The shoulders are relaxed; the trunk, spine and core long. The core is soft; perineum and anus, tongue and eyes, soft and passive.

- **Sit with your legs crossed in front of you**.
- Take your left heel in towards the right buttock bone, keeping the shinbone tight into the thighbone.
- **Place your right foot flat on the floor with the heel against the left ankle, shin vertical, knee up.**
- Take hold of your right shin with both hands. Broadening and flattening your pubic abdomen so the pelvic floor is passively lifted, engage mulabandha. Broadening the ribcrests, suck the solar plexus in, with the abdomen passive, and engage uddiyana-bandha.
- **Press your right foot into the floor, engaging the calf and thigh.**
- Extend your right arm upwards and lengthen your trunk and spine as you look up along your arm.
- **Turning to the right, extend your right arm down to the floor behind you in line with your sacrum.**
- Pushing from your right hand, raise, extend, and look up your left arm to relengthen your trunk
- **Keeping that length in your trunk, wrap your left arm firmly round your right leg.**
- Re-extend the trunk, making your spine and core long.
- **Turn your head gently to the right and look over your shoulder.**

Hold the posture – with your right leg and arm active; aware of the free flow of inhalation and exhalation; abdomen passive, long and hollow; solar plexus sucked in; chest broad and active; pubic abdomen flat and broad; anus soft – until ready to release. Repeat on the other side.

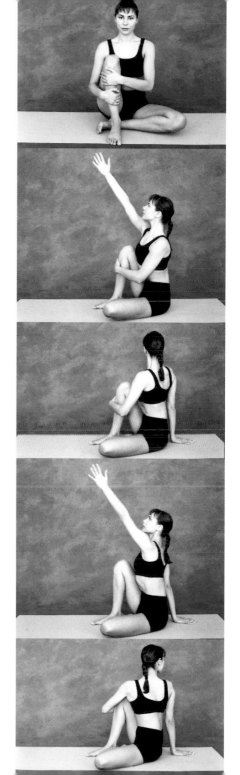

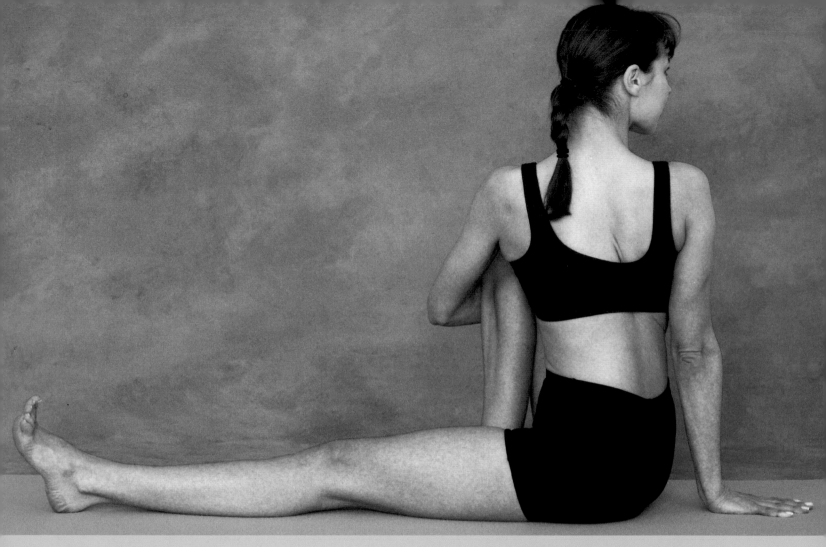

maricyasana

The front leg is kept active, thigh muscles sucking into the bone and pressing the leg down into the floor. The foot of the front leg is engaged – ball broad; inner and front ankle, Achilles tendon and toes long. The foot of the bent leg presses into the floor as an active part of the foundation. The front of the buttock bones and the leading hand and arm are also part of the dynamic of the foundation. The hand of the 'wrapping' arm is kept alive and open. The shoulders are relaxed; the trunk, spine and core long. The core is soft; perineum and anus, tongue and eyes, soft and passive.

- **Sit in dandasana.**
- Bend your right leg and place the foot flat on the floor, touching the inner left thigh with its heel back against the thigh.
- **Engage your left leg, pressing it down into the floor as you suck the thigh muscles into the bone and engage the foot.**
- Take hold of your right shin with both hands. Broadening and flattening your pubic abdomen so the pelvic floor is passively lifted, engage mulabandha. Broadening the ribcrests, suck the solar plexus in with the abdomen passive, and engage uddiyanabandha.
- **Press your right foot into the floor, engaging the calf and thigh.**
- Extend your right arm upwards and lengthen your trunk and spine as you look up along your arm.
- **Turning to the right, extend your right arm down to the floor behind you, in line with your sacrum.**
- Pushing from your right hand, raise, extend, and look up your left arm to relengthen your trunk
- **Keeping that length in your trunk, wrap your left arm firmly round your right leg.**
- Re-extend the trunk, making your spine and core long.
- **Turn your head gently to the right and look over your shoulder.**

Hold the posture – your legs and arms active; aware of the free flow of inhalation and exhalation; abdomen passive, long and hollow; solar plexus sucked in; chest broad and active; pubic abdomen flat and broad; anus soft – until ready to release. Repeat on the other side.

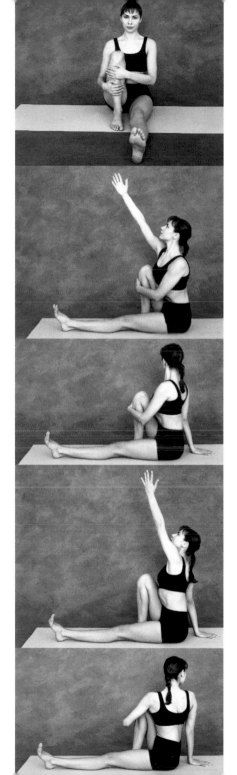

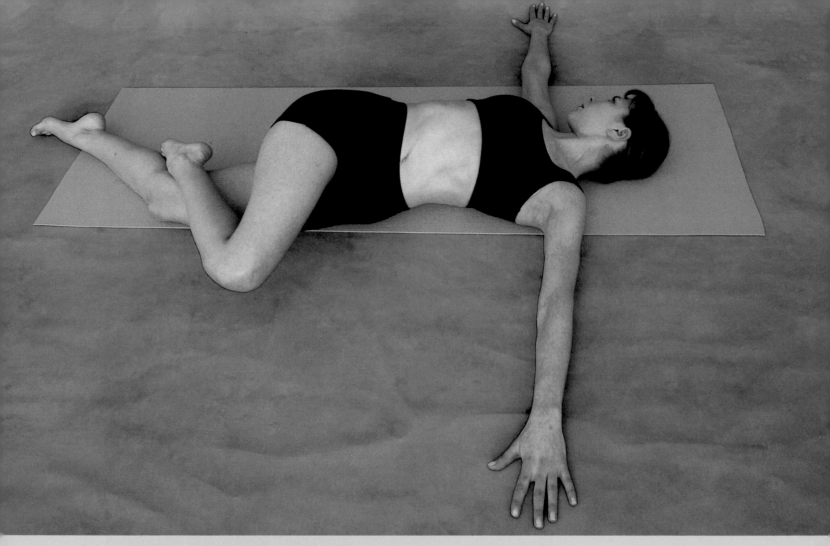

suptaparivritasana

In this posture the whole body is allowed to let go, with the exception of the bandhas. This may not be as easy as it sounds. The line of the lower leg and exact placing of the top foot is arbitrary, let them be wherever complete relaxation becomes easier. If the shoulder opposite the legs cannot stay down by itself, then you can use its arm to ground the shoulder by pressing the palm down and spiralling and lengthening the arm.

- Lie on your back in savasana.
- **Extend your arms out straight from your armpits.**
- Bend your right leg and place its foot flat on the floor by the inside of the left knee.
- **Pressing down with your right foot, lift the pelvis gently off the floor. Tucking your left hip back and under, roll the right hip over to the left, taking the right knee and leg with you.**
- Relax both legs and allow your right foot and leg to find a comfortable position where they can fully let go.
- **Turn your head to the right, extend your arms, press the palms down and spiral and lengthen the arms, bringing the shoulders to the floor.**
- Broadening and flattening your pubic abdomen so the pelvic floor is passively lifted, engage mulabandha. Broadening the ribcrests, suck the solar plexus in, with the abdomen passive, and engage uddiyanabandha.

Hold the posture – with your abdomen passive, long and hollow; solar plexus sucked in; chest broad and active; pubic abdomen flat and broad; anus and core soft; aware of the free flow of inhalation and exhalation – until ready to release. Repeat on the other side.

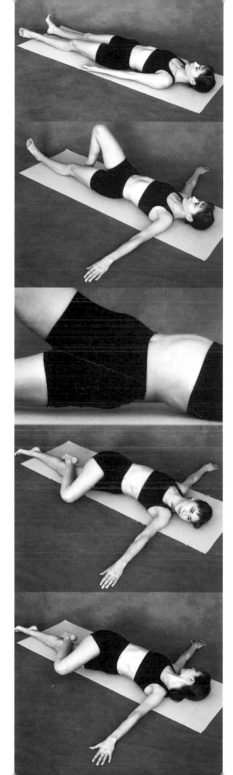

THE TWISTING PRACTICE

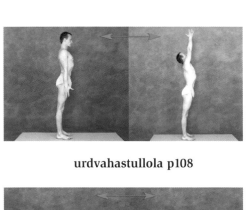

urdvahastullola p108

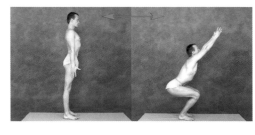

utktullola p108

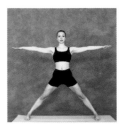

trikonasana p38

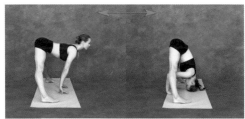

padottanullola p109

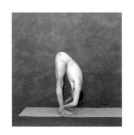

trikonasana p38

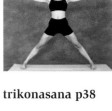

uttanasana p96

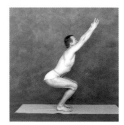

utktasana p96

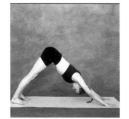

adomukasvanasana p82

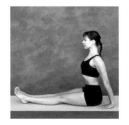

dandasana p40

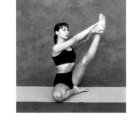

chakrasukasana p25

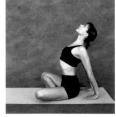

urdvaikapadasana p162

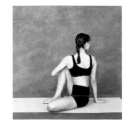

chakrasukasana p25

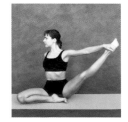

parsvaikapadasana p164

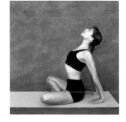

chakrasukasana p25

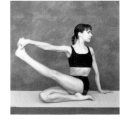

parivritaikapad-asana p166

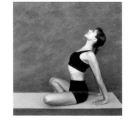

chakrasukasana p25

sukamaricyasana p192

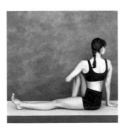 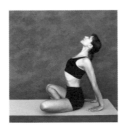 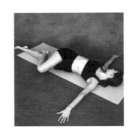 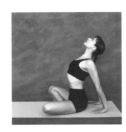 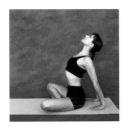

chakrasukasana p25   maricyasana p194   chakrasukasana p25   suptaparixvritasana p196   chakrasukasana p25

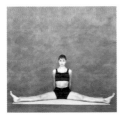 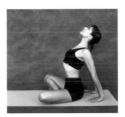 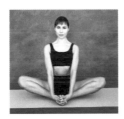 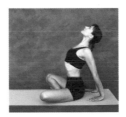 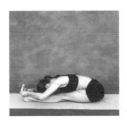

urdvakonasana p176   chakrasukasana p25   urdvabadakonasana p178   chakrasukasana p25   pascimasana p180

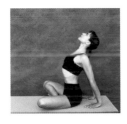 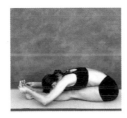 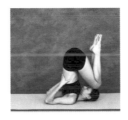 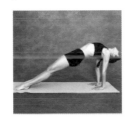 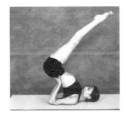

chakrasukasana p25   pascimottanasana p182   purvottanasana p184   ardapindasana p44   ardasarvangasana p70

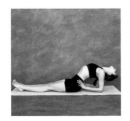 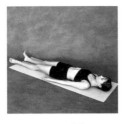 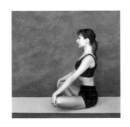

ardamatsyasana p72   savasana p22   sukasana p24

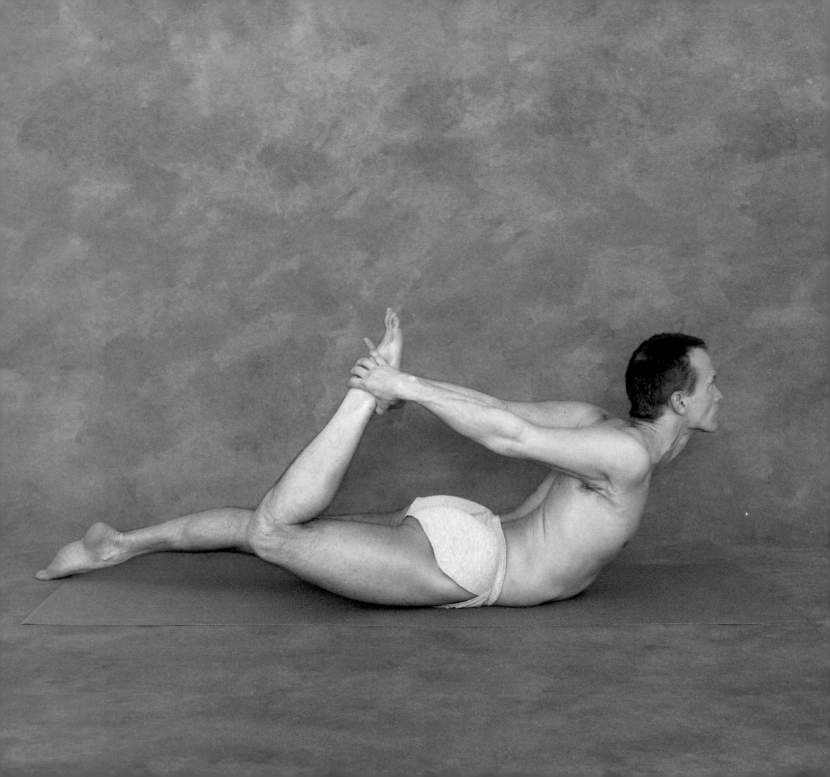

STRENGTHENING THE SPINE

The condition of the spine depends to a great extent on the condition of the back muscles. Both tension and weakness in the back muscles render the spine vulnerable to injury through repetitive stress or sudden shock. When the back muscles have areas of tension, especially embedded habitual patterns that have become the norm, this can disturb the spine in two ways. First, it can create imbalanced lines of force on the vertebrae, destabilizing them. Second, it can create a distorted pattern of weight-bearing that overworks some muscles while others become dormant and atrophy. This can then cause all kinds of back and spinal problems, from undiagnosable pains to slipped and ruptured disks.

When the back carries a lot of tension it is not uncommon for that tension to become a significant weight bearer. The back then fails to distribute the work of weight-bearing evenly and organically throughout its muscles. This can lead to temporary problems when this tension is released. The muscles that ordinarily would and should have been bearing weight have not been. As a result they are not prepared to because they are too weak. This can cause immediate compensatory tension in these and other muscles, due to the release of habitual tension creating new, compensatory tension. To avoid this, the body needs to be strengthened, as well as released from tension. This is a vital consideration in any yoga practice. Too often the focus – overall or on any specific area of the body – is on opening, release and flexibility, with strengthening and stability overlooked. This can cause problems. Besides the possibility of stimulating compensatory tension, it can also lead to overstretching, which weakens the muscles and worse, the ligaments. Overstretched muscles can soon be retuned. Overstretched ligaments are another, often painful, story.

The postures in this lesson are not only flexions of the spine that balance the movement of forward extensions, they also develop deep strength in the lower back and the front of the trunk and pelvis (as well as strengthening the sacroilic joint). Unlike many other backbends, they are quite safe to do – even when the spine is not well trained in forward extensions and rotations and twists. They do not involve extreme movement and the focus is on lifting, rather than bending. Their key is the work in the legs. This work is an extension and expression of the way that the legs have been learning to work in the other postures. However, it can feel very different and is much more challenging to establish and maintain. This challenge must not be given up. If these postures are done without the leg work then they do become unsafe for the back and spine. The legs are used to stabilize the sacrum and pelvis, and to broaden and lengthen the lower back. This protects them, and the vertebrae, from strain and injury. As the legs extend one way out of the pelvis, the spine extends the other. The more the legs extend and lengthen, the more freely and safely will the spine.

ardashalabasana

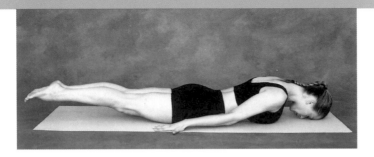

Half-locust teaches the use of the legs in supine backbends and the complementary extension of legs and trunk.

Half-locust strengthens the front trunk muscles, the back and the sacroiliac joints; opens the chest; mobilizes the top spine; develops the legs and feet; and releases the shoulders. Mulabandha stabilizes the lungs and sacrum, while uddiyanabandha protects the lower back.

ardabujangasana

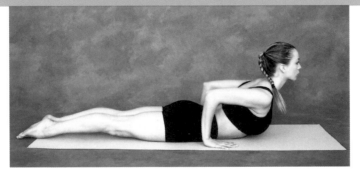

Half-cobra teaches the use of the legs in supine backbends and the complementary extension of legs and trunk. It also teaches the role of the hands and shoulders in opening the chest.

Half-cobra strengthens the front trunk muscles, the back and the sacroiliac joints; opens the chest; mobilizes the top spine; develops the legs and feet; and releases the shoulders. Mulabandha stabilizes the lungs and sacrum, while uddiyanabandha protects the lower back.

shalabasana

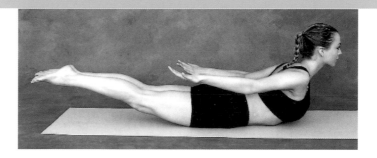

Locust pose teaches the use of the legs in supine backbends and the complementary extension of legs and trunk. It also teaches the role of the arms and shoulders in opening the chest.

Locust pose strengthens the front trunk muscles, the back and the sacroiliac joints; opens the chest; mobilizes the top spine; develops the legs and feet; and releases the shoulders. Mulabandha stabilizes the lungs and sacrum, while uddiyanabandha protects the lower back.

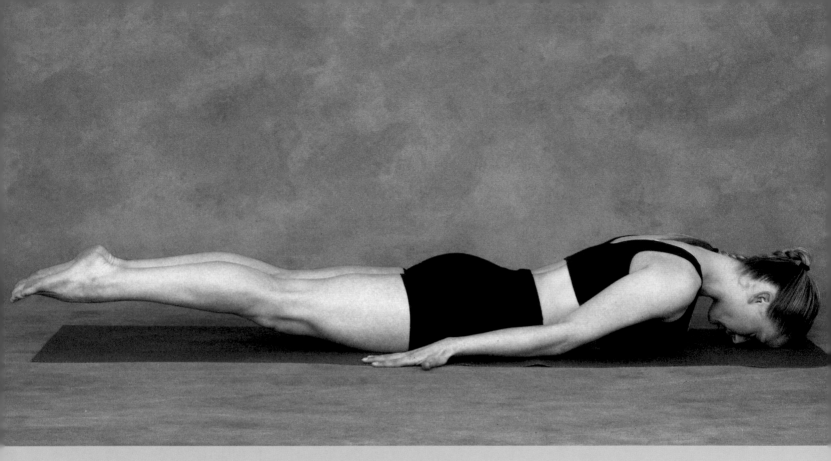

ardashalabasana

The legs must be kept fully engaged throughout. The thigh muscles are sucked into the bone, which requires the support of the feet. The balls of the feet are broad, the inner ankles pressing against each other and away from the body; the front ankles and inner edges of the feet long. The internal spiral of the feet and legs are emphasized to keep the buttocks and sacroiliac joints from tightening, and the sacrum and lower back broad. The external spiral of the feet and legs are emphasized to stabilize the legs and pelvis. The forehead is activated against the floor, with the chin on the chest in jalandhara-bandha. The shoulders are actively rolled back, away from the ears, to open the chest. They are supported by the spirallic action of the arms and hands. The lower back and buttocks are kept passive and soft. It is not important how high the feet lift, they can just clear the floor. What is important is that the legs are kept engaged, strong and straight.

- Lie face-down on the floor, arms beside you.
- Lifting one foot at a time off the floor, stretch your legs back out of the pelvis, making them long.
- **Press the inner edges of your feet together and broaden the balls of your feet as you lengthen the inner and front ankles. Suck your thigh muscles into the bones, making the legs long and strong. Keep your buttocks passive.**
- Roll your shoulders back and tuck your chin in.
- Press your hands into the floor, palms down, and spiral your arms.
- **Raise your feet off the floor, keeping your legs straight.**

Hold the posture – with your legs and feet, arms and hands engaged; abdomen passive, long and hollow; solar plexus sucked in; chest broad and active; pubic abdomen flat and broad; anus and core soft; aware of the free flow of inhalation and exhalation – until ready to release.

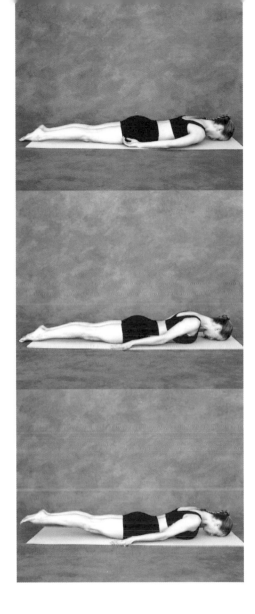

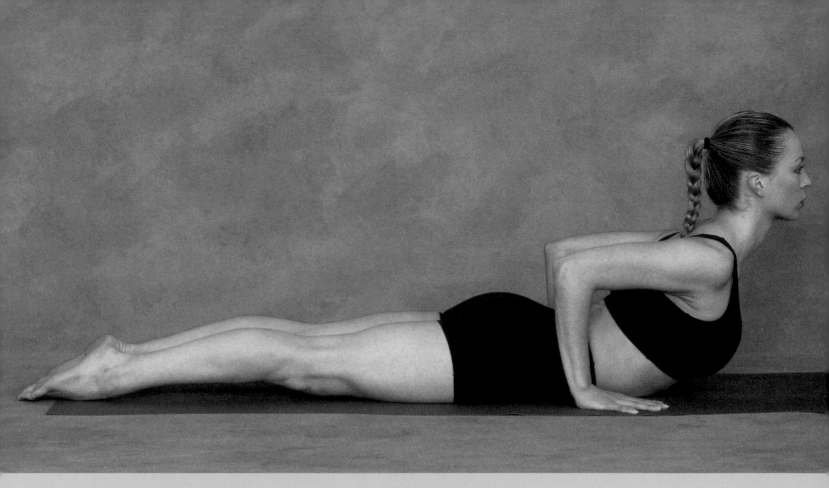

ardabujangasana

The legs must be kept fully engaged throughout. The thigh muscles are sucked into the bone, which requires the support of the feet. The balls of the feet are broad, the inner ankles pressing against each other and away from the body; the front ankles and inner edges of the feet long. The internal spiral of the feet and legs are emphasized to keep the buttocks and sacroiliac joints from tightening, and the sacrum and lower back broad. The external spiral of the feet and legs are emphasized to stabilize the legs and pelvis. The shoulders are actively rolled back, away from the ears, to open the chest. They are supported by the spirallic action of the arms and hands. The lower back and buttocks are kept passive and soft. Do not lift the ribcrests off the floor. Make sure you place the hands close to the hips, not forward by the shoulders.

- Lie face-down on the floor, arms beside you.
- Lifting one foot at a time off the floor, stretch your legs back out of the pelvis, making them long.
- **Press the inner edges of your feet together and broaden the balls of your feet as you lengthen the inner and front ankles. Suck your thigh muscles into the bones, making the legs long and strong. Keep your buttocks passive.**
- Roll your shoulders back and tuck your chin in.
- **Bend your arms and place the palms on the floor near the hips so that although the fingers can lengthen along the floor, the heel of the hand is not able to make contact with it.**
- Leading from the base of your skull to your chin, lift the head up and look forwards.
- **Pressing your hands into the floor, raise the top chest off the floor so that the heels of your hands ground down into the floor and the ribcrests remain grounded on the floor.**

When you become comfortable in this position you can release the hands and stretch them back, parallel to the floor.

Hold the posture – with your legs and feet, arms and hands engaged; abdomen passive, long and hollow; solar plexus sucked in; chest broad and active; pubic abdomen flat and broad; anus and core soft; aware of the free flow of inhalation and exhalation – until ready to release.

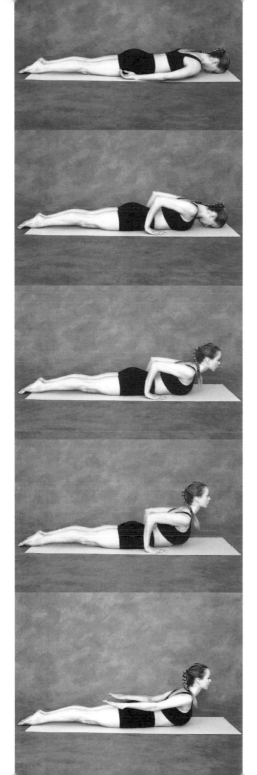

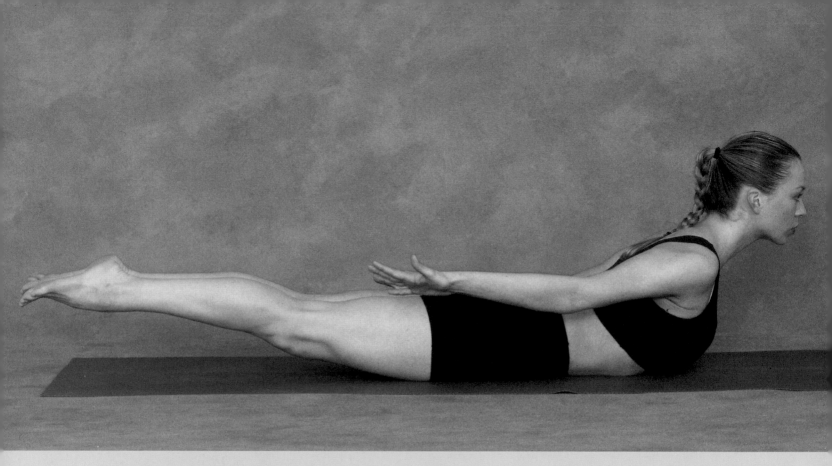

shalabasana

The legs must be kept fully engaged throughout. The thigh muscles are sucked into the bone, which requires the support of the feet. The balls of the feet are broad, the inner ankles pressing against each other and away from the body; the front ankles and inner edges of the feet long. The internal spiral of the feet and legs are emphasized to keep the buttocks and sacroiliac joints from tightening, and the sacrum and lower back broad. The external spirals of the feet and legs are emphasized to stabilize the legs and pelvis. The shoulders are actively rolled back, away from the ears, to open and lift the chest. They are supported by the spirallic action of the arms and hands extending backwards. The lower back and buttocks are kept passive and soft. When you complete the pose by lifting your head, lead from the base of the skull to the chin and keep the neck soft and comfortable.

- Lie face-down on the floor, arms beside you.
- Lifting one foot at a time off the floor, stretch your legs back out of the pelvis, making them long.
- **Press the inner edges of your feet together and broaden the balls of your feet as you lengthen the inner and front ankles. Suck your thigh muscles into the bones, making the legs long and strong. Keep your buttocks passive.**
- Roll your shoulders back and tuck your chin in.
- Press your hands into the floor and spiral your arms.
- **Raise your feet off the floor, keeping your legs straight.**
- Raise your palms off the floor and stretch your arms parallel to the floor with the hands alive. Lift your chin to lengthen the front of your spine, and look forwards.
- **Raise your legs as high as you can without bending them.**
- Lift up onto your ribcrests and extend from your navel to your chin.

Hold the posture – with your legs and feet, arms and hands engaged; abdomen passive, long and hollow; solar plexus sucked in; chest broad and active; pubic abdomen flat and broad; anus and core soft; aware of the free flow of inhalation and exhalation – until ready to release.

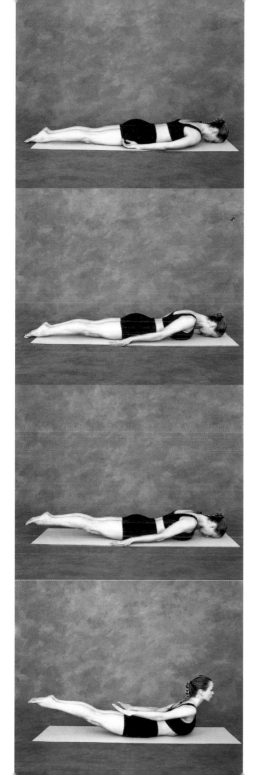

THE STRENGTHENING PRACTICE

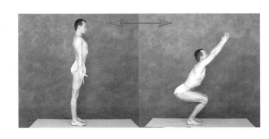

urdvahastullola p108

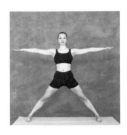

utktullola p108

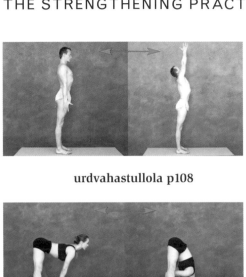

trikonasana p38

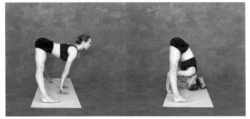

padottanullola p109

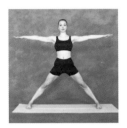

trikonasana p38

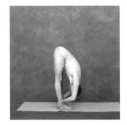

uttanasana p96

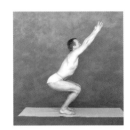

utktasana p96

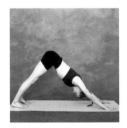

adomukasvan-asana p82

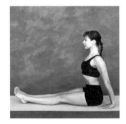

dandasana p40

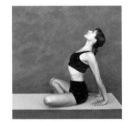

chakrasukasana p25

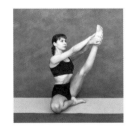

urdvaikapadasana p162

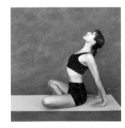

chakrasukasana p25

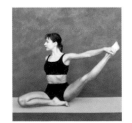

parsvaikapad-asana p164

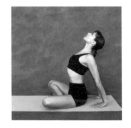

chakrasukasana p25

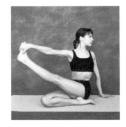

parivritaikapad-asana p166

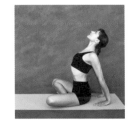

chakrasukasana p25

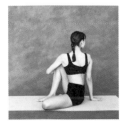

sukamaricyasana p192

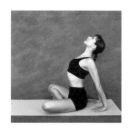 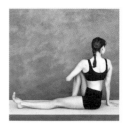 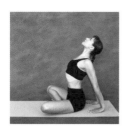 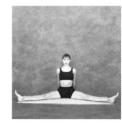 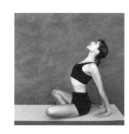

chakrasukasana p25   maricyasana p194   chakrasukasana p25   urdvakonasana p176   chakrasukasana p25

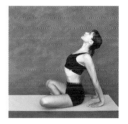 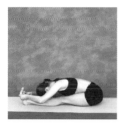 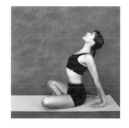 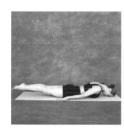 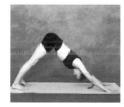

urdvabadakonasana p178   chakrasukasana p25   pascimasana p180   chakrasukasana p25   ardashalabasana p204

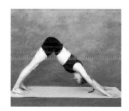 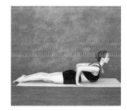 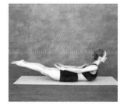 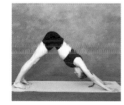 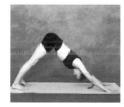

adomukasvan-asana p82   ardabujangasana p206   adomukasvan-asana p82   shalabasana p208   adomukasvan-asana p82

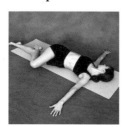 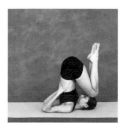 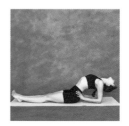 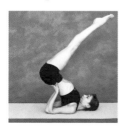 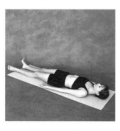

suptaparivritasana p196   ardapindasana p44   ardasarvangasana p70   ardamatsyasana p72   savasana p22

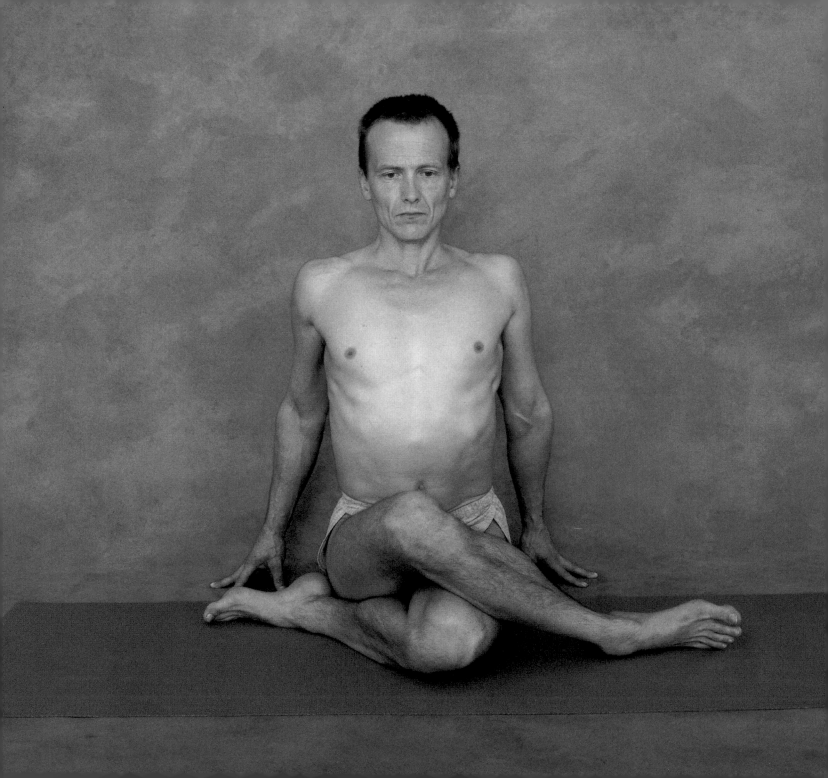

THE ART OF STILLNESS

Yoga is not about transcending, destroying or dismantling the mind. It is about opening to the more subtle, innate capacities of the mind: allowing these capacities to play their role in the way we live our lives. The conventional mind is a divisive, fragmented one: based on dividing this from that, categorizing these as apart from those. It is based upon the implementation of duality. It is this conventional mind that yoga, like all spiritual practices, is designed to liberate us from. However, the conventional, categorising mind with its labels, compartments, statistics and formulae is necessary to the survival of the human organism. Without it we could neither hunt nor farm, weave nor sew, design nor build. We would be a vulnerable biped, with neither the physical skills of speed, camouflage or built-in weaponry, nor the mental skills of anticipation, preparation and fabrication to utilize for our survival. We would not exist.

Somehow, however, we have allowed our analytical, rational mind to outstrip its brief and usurp the functions of other aspects of our intelligence. Reason may be perfect for designing and building a house; it is woefully inadequate for navigating affairs of the heart, or setting us a course in life capable of satisfying us. Yoga gives us the opportunity, indeed demands, that we awaken and develop different modes of intelligence. Nevertheless, in the beginning, we have to approach it with a mode of intelligence that is greatly inadequate to it – reason.

The various aspects of yoga are not inherently separate from each other. Attitude, orientation, posture, breathing, internalization, concentration, contemplation and absorption are not contained within a linear relationship. This is not to say that they cannot be, and often are, accessed in a linear manner. It simply means that a linear relationship is not their essential one. They are more like facets of a diamond: each one opening into the same internal space, each one affording a different access and offering a different flavour. So it is that schools of yoga have evolved that focus almost exclusively on this aspect or that of the practice. Bhakti Yoga, for example, can be seen as a refined and focused development of the fifth orientation: devotion. Jnana Yoga can be seen as a refined and focused development of the fourth orientation: self-enquiry. Hatha yoga can be seen as a refined and focused development of the third orientation: passion.

Posture is not yoga posture without the five attitudes and the five orientations. It is not yoga posture without awareness of the breath. Pranayama is not simply awareness of the breath. It transcends the distinction between inhalation and exhalation, breather and breath. In doing so, it dislocates the conventional mind and readies us for meditation by internalizing us to the activity of our soul. The unravelling of the activity of our soul that occurs in meditation is a natural consequence of this internalization.

Therefore, the crucible of ashtanga yoga practice is asana: the postures. To the extent that they free the body from tension, they generate a joyful steadiness. As this joyful steadiness stabilizes, the body transcends its experiential dualities. As this occurs, the sense of the physical body evaporates and awareness is left with only the spontaneous rhythm of the breath. As the breather comes closer and closer to the breath, its dualities – of inhale and exhale, action and rest – are also transcended. This undermines and disempowers the dualistic activity of the mind. The mind is then pulled away from the realm of memory and the senses. Going deeper into itself it encounters its inner activity. This is the response of the mind to traces left over from unresolved past actions: karmic imprints. The purpose of meditation is to resolve these karmic imprints, and free us from the binding chains of our karma. Then we can live life freely and fully, in honest and honourable expression of its beauty and bounty.

All of this occurs quite naturally within the stillness of asana or yoga posture. Which, of course, depends upon the contextual support of the five attitudes and orientations. Stillness in asana, however, is not automatic. Many postures are too complex and demanding to permit the sustained stillness that meditation requires. For this reason a whole range of sitting postures has been developed. They all permit the spine to express its innate verticality effortlessly, from the stability of a base made up of the pelvis and the legs. The differences between these postures is mainly one of the arrangement of the legs.

It is not enough to shake ourselves up through our practice and then let the flotsam and jetsam settle back again into their old or more hidden places. We must take the opportunity that the internal shakedown of our dynamic practice offers. We must resolve what has been released. This requires sustained stillness. At the end of our yoga posture practice, then, we take a sitting posture. After the dynamic aspect of our practice, this allows us to be still. Having used the more active postures to challenge and release our limitations, we can now resolve them. This we do in the light of the awareness that becomes possible within sustained stillness.

There is a method to sitting in sustained stillness. It is a direct continuation of the method of the more dynamic yoga postures. First it involves creating stability by establishing a safe and secure base. Equally, it requires comfort – a complete freedom from tension. To the extent that our body still carries tension, we will find the internalization required of meditation very elusive. This internalization cannot be imposed by the will. To try to do so simply reduces meditation to psychic manipulation. It is possible to become very skilful at psychic manipulation and generate fascinating states of consciousness, and impose stillness and silence on the mind. This has nothing to do with sensitivity, honesty, openness, focus, or generosity. It has even less to do with self-enquiry. It is a subtle form of aggression which, while it may lead to the development of exotic, fascinating and charismatic skills and powers, does not lead to the heart of yoga. However, it is possible to release physical tension internally, from the stillness of a sitting posture. This is how Zen works. Tension in the body is a manifestation of psychological resistance and crystallization. Through allowing ourselves to become familiar with and to become one with the neurotic activity of our mind we resolve it. As the neuroses of the mind are resolved, their physical counterparts are also. So the dynamic yoga postures do not work alone. The sitting postures also greatly contribute to freeing the body from tension, by opening the mind.

When taking a sitting posture within which we wish to access the depths of our mind, we take the steps outlined overleaf. Take your time over each step. If you are really honest you will probably find that it takes days or weeks to master each step. Don't be impatient. Remember the hare and the tortoise. Yoga practice is the same. Careful and deliberate application of each step, step by simple step is the way forward. Each of these steps prepares for the one that follows. If you rush on to one before its precursor has been established, each step will become more and more elusive. If this is your style of practice you will probably have to indulge in all kinds of undermining self-deceptions to convince yourself that you are doing something worthwhile. Don't waste your energy. Be sensitive, honest, open, focussed and generous to yourself. You have the time. Cultivate the patience.

STEP ONE: ESTABLISHING THE BASE

Sit on the floor, or a raised support, in an upright position with a triangular base formed by the shins and the buttock bones. The front edges of the buttock bones should be on the front edge of your support, with the hip-bones slightly forward of the buttock bones. Both shinbones should be securely supported by the floor. Relax all the muscles in your feet and legs, including ankles, knees and hip sockets.

STEP TWO: RELAXING YOUR BODY

Keeping your waist long, chest lifted and open, release all your body muscles systematically and repeatedly – especially shoulders, jaw and face – until you can feel your whole body melting effortlessly down to your base and into the floor.

STEP THREE: RELAXING YOUR CORE

Focusing especially on your perineum and the root of your tongue, release your core fully, continuously checking the quality of your anus, eyes, ears, brain, tongue, palate, anus and perineum.

STEP FOUR: RELEASING YOUR SPINE

Within the downward softening of your outer body and the inward opening of your core, feel your spine effortlessly expressing its inherent elevation out of the pelvis as a flowing upwards from the perineum to the brain, like a fountain rather than a fixed, solid object.

STEP FIVE: TUNING INTO YOUR POSTURE

Tune into the dynamic of your posture created by your spine vertically expressing itself within the softening of your outer body and your core: especially the quality of perineum and tongue root.

STEP SIX: TUNING INTO YOUR EXHALATION

Within your awareness of the dynamic of your posture – rooted in continuous awareness of perineum and tongue root – give the support of your attentiveness to your exhalation, ensuring that it is a spontaneous letting go and that you are not pushing the air out, however subtly. Allow your exhalation to fulfil itself naturally and fully without any imposition upon it by your inhalation, and without attempting to prolong, deepen or maximize your exhalation at all.

STEP SEVEN: TUNING INTO YOUR INHALATION

Within your awareness of the dynamic of your posture – rooted in continuous awareness of perineum and tongue root – give the support of your attentiveness to your inhalation, ensuring that it is allowed to originate itself naturally without any imposition upon it by your intent or by habit, and without imposing an unnatural pause after your exhalation, but allowing whatever pause arises naturally to be.

STEP EIGHT: TUNING INTO YOUR BREATH

Within your awareness of the dynamic of your posture and continuous awareness of the passive quality of your core, from the perineum to the brain, feel the spontaneous flow of your breathing filling and emptying you. Without taking account of either the exhalation or the inhalation as such, allow your awareness to be taken fully by the rhythm of your breath. Allow your awareness to oscillate between the fullness and emptiness of your breath, between the presence and absence of your self, between your finite and your infinite nature.

STEP NINE: TUNING IN

As you sit within the comfortable stability of your breathing, be present to all that arises in your awareness without reaction – neither moving towards the pleasant and intriguing, nor moving away from the unpleasant and unwelcome. Simply be one with the activity of your mind, allowing it to play itself out freely and fully with neither help nor hindrance from you.

Stay with this process as long as you like. Make the transition to everyday consciousness by eventually bringing your attention to bear on the data flowing through your senses from your environment. Sit comfortably and easily within the re-externalization of your awareness until you are ready to release the posture. Lie down for a moment before taking up the activity of your life. Initially these steps are best learned and applied in a linear manner. As your familiarity with them deepens you can apply them in groups, and eventually all together.

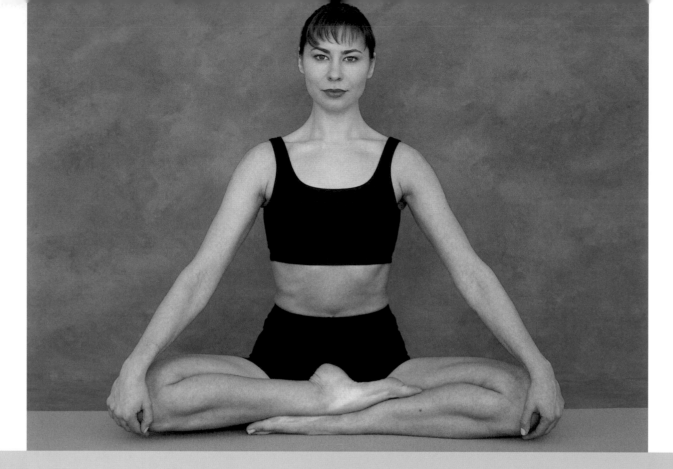

siddhasana

Sit with the support of a secure triangular base made up of the front edge of your buttock bones and your shins. The trunk and the spine should be vertical – use supports if you need to. Keep the shoulders relaxed with the trunk and spine long, core soft. Don't move for itches, aches or other distracting irritations. They are just the mind trying to find a way back to its habit of continuously changing activity and stimulus. Let go of any impulse to move as soon as you are aware of it. If you make a genuine commitment to sit still and find your way to the heart of your breath and the depths of your mind, there is no need to fight with yourself and impose any draconian discipline. If you do have a real commitment, and are not simply playing games with yourself, then as soon as you notice that your mind has wandered off the point, it will come back. This does not have to be enforced. If it does require force, take a closer look at your intentions. If you don't really intend to meditate, but just want to make it look like you are, don't waste your time.

- Sit with your legs relaxed in front of you.
- **Draw your feet in towards your pubic bones.**
- Separate your knees and place one heel back against the pubic bone or the pelvic floor.
- **Place the other heel on top of the first, making the top foot secure.**
- Use your hands to bring you forward onto the front edges of your buttock bones.
- **Flatten the palms down into the floor at the sides of your buttocks and engage your arms to lift your trunk upwards, keeping the pelvis grounded.**
- Place your hands, wrists or forearms on your knees. Keep the hands, arms and shoulders completely relaxed.

Hold the posture – with your abdomen relaxed, chest lifted – and begin to take the steps outlined on the previous pages.

If you find that your head and chest are dropping forwards and down and your lower back is rounding, you need to use some support. Place a book, block or folded rug under your buttock bones.

If you still feel like you will collapse, place your hands behind you and use them and your arms to help keep the spine vertical.

If you cannot relax your hip sockets completely because your shins and knees are not supported, place a book, block or folded rug under each knee.

If you cannot comfortably place one heel on top of the other, place the second foot just in front of the first.

If this is not possible, sit in sukasana with the knees wide apart.

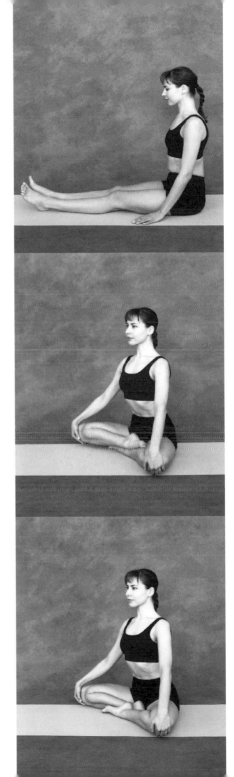

THE FULL PRACTICE

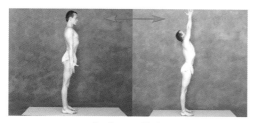

urdvahastullola p108

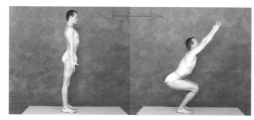

utktullola p108

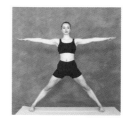

trikonasana p38

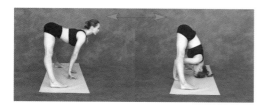

padottanullola p109

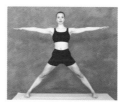

trikonasana p38

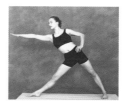

parsvasana p118

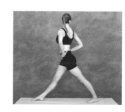

parivritasana p120

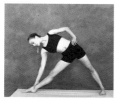

salambatrikon-
asana p122

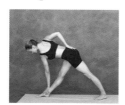

salambaparivritatri-
konasana p124

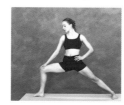

salambaparsvavira-
badrasana p134

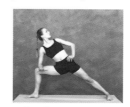

salambaparsva-
konasana p136

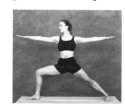

parsvavirabad-
rasana p138

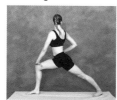

salambavira-
badrasana p148

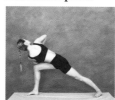

namaskarparsva-
konasana p150

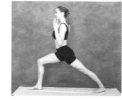

hastavirabad-
rasana p152

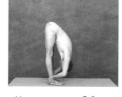

uttanasana p96

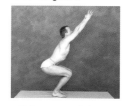

utktasana p96

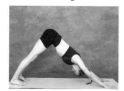

adomukasvan-
asana p82

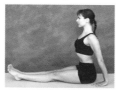

dandasana p40

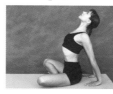

chakrasukasana p25

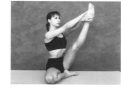

urdvaikapadasana
p162

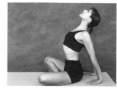

chakrasukasana p25

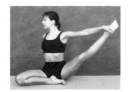 parsvaikapad-asana p164

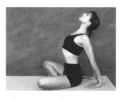 chakrasukasana p25

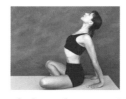 parivritaikapad-asana p166

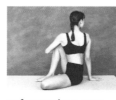 chakrasukasana p25

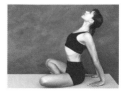 sukamaricyasana p192

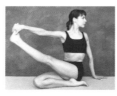 chakrasukasana p25

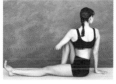 maricyasana p194

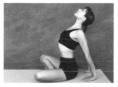 chakrasukasana p25

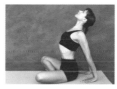 urdvakonasana p176

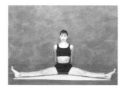 chakrasukasana p25

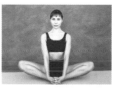 urdvabadakonasana p178

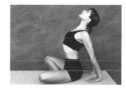 chakrasukasana p25

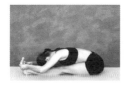 pascimasana p180

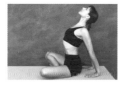 chakrasukasana p25

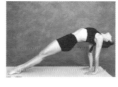 pascimottanasana p182

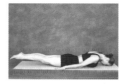 purvottanasana p184

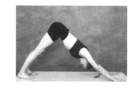 ardashalabasana p204

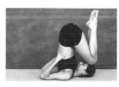 adomukasvan-asana p82

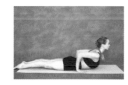 ardabujangasana p206

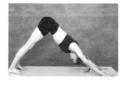 adomukasvan-asana p82

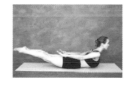 shalabasana p208

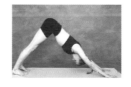 adomukasvan-asana p82

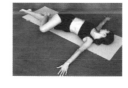 suptaparivritasana p196

ardapindasana p44

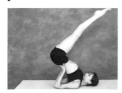 ardasarvangasana asana p70

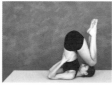 ardapindasana p44

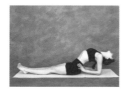 ardamatsyasana p72

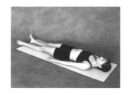 savasana p22

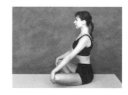 sukasana p24

EXTRA SHORTER PRACTICES

THE BACKBEND PRACTICE

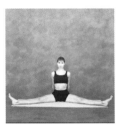

urdvakonasana
p176

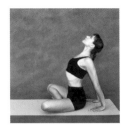

chakrasukasana p25

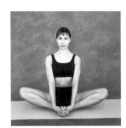

urdvabadakon-
asana p178

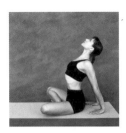

chakrasukasana p25

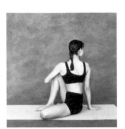

sukamaricyasana
p192

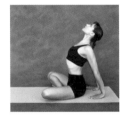

chakrasukasana p25

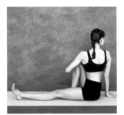

maricyasana p194

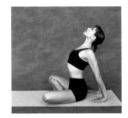

chakrasukasana p25

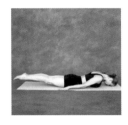

ardashalabasana
p204

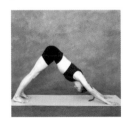

adomukasvan-
asana p82

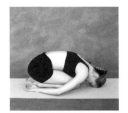

balasana p26

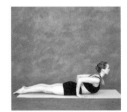

ardabujangasana
p206

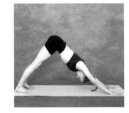

adomukasvan-
asana p82

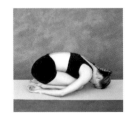

balasana p26

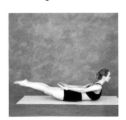

shalabasana p208

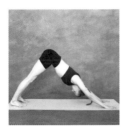

adomukasvan-
asana p82

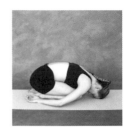

balasana p26

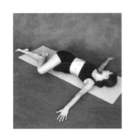

suptaparivritasana
p196

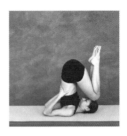

ardapindasana p44

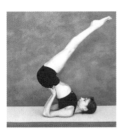

ardasarvangasana
p70

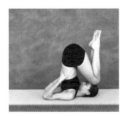

ardapindasana p44

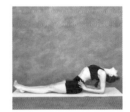

ardamatsyasana
p72

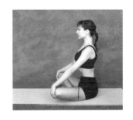

savasana p22

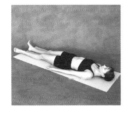

sukasana p24

THE QUIETENING PRACTICE

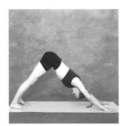

adomukasvan-
asana p82

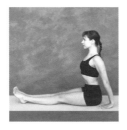

dandasana p40

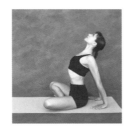

chakrasukasana p25

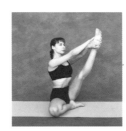

urdvaikapadasana
p162

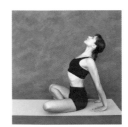

chakrasukasana p25

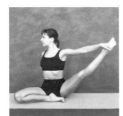

parsvaikapad-
asana p164

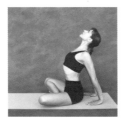

chakrasukasana p25

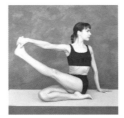

parivritaikapad-
asana p166

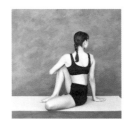

chakrasukasana p25

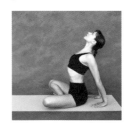

sukamaricyasana
p192

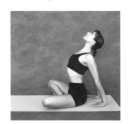

chakrasukasana p25

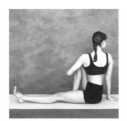

maricyasana p194

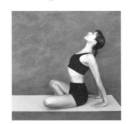

chakrasukasana p25

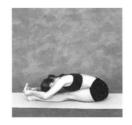

pascimasana p180

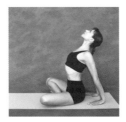

chakrasukasana p25

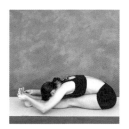

pascimottanasana
p182

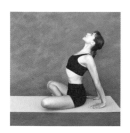

chakrasukasana p25

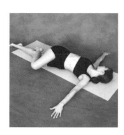

suptaparivrit-
asana p196

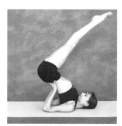

ardapindasana p44

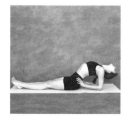

ardasarvangasana
p70

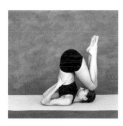

ardapindasana p44

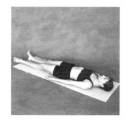

ardamatsyasana p72

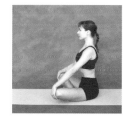

savasana p22

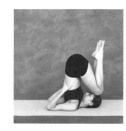

sukasana p24

index

Page numbers in **bold** refer to main entries for postures, including details of the involvement of the bandhas and full step-by-step instructions.

Page numbers in *italics* refer to practice sequences.

abdominal lock *see* uddiyanabandha
adomukasvanasana **80**, **82–3**, **91**
  backbend practice *222*
  breath practice *110*
  downwards-dog practice *84*
  extension practice *186*
  full practice *220*, *221*
  leg practice *98*
  lunge practice *141*
  quietening practice *224*
  raised leg practice *168*
  standing practice *126*
  strengthening practice *210*, *211*
  twisting practice *198*
  warrior practice *155*
ahimsa (sensitivity) 3
all-fours pose *see* svanasana
anatomical postures 157
aparigraha (generosity) 3, 4
ardabujangasana **202**, **206–7**, *211*, *221*,
  222
ardamatsyasana **69**, **72–3**
  backbend practice *223*
  bandha practice *74*
  breath practice *111*
  downwards-dog practice *84*
  extension practice *187*
  full practice *221*
  leg practice *98*

lunge practice *141*
quietening practice *225*
raised leg practice *169*
standing practice *127*
strengthening practice *211*
twisting practice *199*
warrior practice *155*
ardapindasana **37**, **44–5**
  backbend practice *223*
  bandha practice *74*
  breath practice *111*
  core practice *56*
  downwards-dog practice *84*
  extension practice *187*
  foundation practice *46*
  full practice *221*
  leg practice *98*
  lunge practice *141*
  quietening practice *225*
  raised leg practice *169*
  standing practice *127*
  strengthening practice *211*
  twisting practice *199*
  warrior practice *155*
ardasarvangasana **67–8**, **70–1**, **93**
  backbend practice *223*
  bandha practice *74*
  breath practice *111*
  downwards-dog practice *84*

extension practice *187*
full practice *221*
leg practice *98*
lunge practice *141*
quietening practice *225*
raised leg practice *169*
standing practice *127*
strengthening practice *211*
twisting practice *199*
warrior practice *155*
ardashalabasana **202**, **204–5**, *211*, *221*,
  222
arduttanasana **90**, **97**
arms 66, 77–9, 158
asanas (yoga postures) 6
  breathing 8–9, 101, 216–17
  categories 157
  context 3–5, 8
  core 7, 49, 216
  'done fully'/'done in correct manner'
    129–30
  dynamic *see* bandhas
  foundation 7, 31
  general instructions 8–12, 14
  role in relaxation 17
  stillness 213–17
  see also individually by name eg
    sukasana
ashtanga (eight limbs) 5, 8, 213

asteya (openness) 3–4
attitudes (yama) 3–5, 8, 17, 213, 214

back & spine 157, 171, 189, 201, 216
backbend practice 222–3
balasana **21**, **26–7**
  basis for adomukasvanasana 83
  in practice sequences 28, 46, 56, 74
bandhas (dynamic) 7–8, 59–60, 65–6
  bandha practice 74
  jalandharabandha 58, 61, 66
  mulabandha 58, 64–5, 66
  spirallic dynamic 65–6, 78–9, 87–8, 113, 129, 143–4
  uddiyanabandha 58, 62–3, 66
  see also parts of body engaged eg legs
bhakti yoga 213
bhramacharya (focus) 3, 4
breath & breathing 6, 8–9, 61, 62–3, 101, 216–17
  pranayama 3, 5, 8, 17, 213–17
breath practice 110–11

chakrasukasana **25**, 168–9, 186–7, 198–9, 210–11, 220–1, 222, 224
child pose see balasana
cobbler poses see suptabadakonasana; urdvabadakonasana
cobra, half- see ardabujangasana
commitment (sauca) 3, 4
core 7, 49, 216
core practice 56
corpse pose see savasana

dandasana **34–5**, **40–1**, **81**, **92**
  bandha practice 74
  basis for other postures 185, 195
  breath practice 111
  core practice 56
  downwards-dog practice 84
  extension practice 186
  foundation practice 46
  full practice 220
  leg practice 98
  lunge practice 141
  quietening practice 224
  raised leg practice 168
  standing practice 127
  strengthening practice 210
  twisting practice 198
  warrior practice 155
devotion (pranidhana) 3, 4–5
dharana (meditative concentration) 5, 8
dhyana (meditative contemplation) 5, 8
dog pose see svanasana
downwards-dog pose see adomukasvanasana
downwards-dog practice 84
dualism 17
dynamic see bandhas
dynamic sequences see padottanullola; tadottanullola; urdvahastullola; utktullola

easy pose see sukasana
easy rotation see sukamaricyasana
easy wheel pose see chakrasukasana
edge, the 10
eight limbs (ashtanga) 5, 8, 213

embryo pose see ardapindasana
enthusiasm (tapas) 4
extension, forward see pascimottanasana
extension, one-leg-forward see pascimasana
extension practice 186–7

feet 31, 65–6, 87–8, 129, 143–4, 157
fierce pose see utktasana
fish, half- see ardamatsyasana
five attitudes & five orientations (yama & niyama) 3–5, 8, 17, 213, 214
focus (bhramacharya) 3, 4
forward extension see pascimottanasana
foundation 7, 31
foundation practice 46
full practice 220–1

gazing pose see urdvapadottanasa
generosity (aparigraha) 3, 4

half-cobra see ardabujangasana
half-fish see ardamatsyasana
half locust see ardashalabasana
half-shoulderstand see ardasarvangasana
hands 31, 65–6, 77–9
hastabalasana **21**
hastatrikonasana **39**
  basis for other postures 119, 121, 123, 125, 135, 137, 149, 151, 153
hastavirabadrasana **147**, **152–3**, 155, 220

hatha yoga
  approach to practice 3–5, 6–8
  general instructions 8–12, 14
  meaning, purpose & function 1, 6
  stillness 213–17
head-raised pose see arduttanasana
honesty (satya) 3

injury prevention 9, 10

jalandharabandha 58, 61, 66
jnana yoga 213

leg practice 98
leg-stretch pose see padottanasana
legs 66, 87–8, 113, 129, 143–4, 157–8,
  201
locks see bandhas
locust, half- see ardashalabasana
locust pose see shalabasana
lunge practice 140–1
lunge, supported see
  salambaparsvakonasana
lunging salute see
  namaskarparsvakonasana
lying twist see suptaparivritasana

maricyasana **190**, **194–5**, *199*, *211*, *221*,
  222, *224*
meditation 5, 8, 213–17
meditative absorption (samadhi) 5, 8
meditative concentration (dharana) 5, 8
meditative contemplation (dhyana) 5, 8
meditative internalization (pratyahara)
  5, 8

mind
  dualities 17
  stillness 213–17
mountain pose 103, 104, **107**
mulabandha 58, 64–5, 66

namaskarparsvakonasana **146**, **150–1**,
  155, *220*
net supporting regulator see jalandharabandha
niyama (orientations) 3–5, 8, 17, 213, 214
non-violence 3

one-leg-forward extension see
  pascimasana
opening pose see purvottanasana
openness (asteya) 3–4
orientations (niyama) 3–5, 8, 17, 213, 214

padottanasana **89**, **94–5**, *98*, 105
padottanullola **105**, **109**
  in practice sequences *110*, *126*, *140*,
    154, *168*, *186*, *198*, *210*, *220*
pain 9, 10
parivritaikapadasana **161**, **166–7**, *169*,
  186, *198*, *210*, *221*, *224*
parivritasana **115**, **120–1**, *126*, *140*,
  154, *220*
parsvaikapadasana **160**, **164–5**, *169*,
  186, *198*, *210*, *221*, *224*
parsvasana **114**, **118–19**, *126*, 129, *140*,
  154, *220*
parsvavirabadrasana **133**, **138–9**, *140*,
  154, *220*
pascimasana **173**, **180–1**, *187*, *199*,

211, *221*, *224*
pascimottanasana **174**, **182–3**, *187*,
  199, *221*, *225*
Patanjili 3, 6, 8
pelvis & pelvic floor 49, 51, 64–5, 113,
  129, 143–4
physiological postures 157
postures see asanas; individual postures
  by name eg sukasana
practice
  approach 3–5, 6–8
  general instructions 8–12, 14
practice sequences 11–12
  backbend 222–3
  bandha 74
  breath 110–11
  core 56
  downwards-dog 84
  extension 186–7
  foundation 46
  full 220–1
  leg 98
  lunge 140–1
  quietening 224–5
  raised leg 168–9
  relaxation 28
  standing 126–7
  strengthening 210–11
  twisting 198–9
  warrior 154–5
pranayama (yoga breathing) 3, 5, 8, 17,
  213–17
pranidhana (devotion) 3, 4–5
pratyahara (meditative internalization)
  5, 8

purvottanasana **175**, **184–5**, *187*, *199*, *221*, *225*

quietening practice *224–5*

raised-leg pose *see* urdvaikapadasana
raised leg practice *168–9*
reaching pose *see* parsvasana
reclining cobbler *see*
    suptabadakonasana
regenerating postures 157
regulators *see* bandhas
relaxation 17, 216
relaxation postures *see* balasana;
    hastabalasana; savasana; sukasana
relaxation practice *28*
resistance 10
restructuring postures 157
revolving triangle *see*
    salambaparivritatrikonasana
root regulator/root lock *see*
    mulabandha
rotation, easy *see* sukamaricyasana
rotation, seated *see* maricyasana
rotations 189

safety 9, 10
salambaparivritatrikonasana **117**,
    124–5, *126*, *140*, *154*, *220*
salambaparsvakonasana **132**, **136–7**,
    140, *154*, *220*
salambaparsvavirabadrasana **131**,
    134–5, *140*, *154*, *220*
salambatrikonasana **116**, **122–3**, *126*,
    140, *154*, *220*

salambavirabadrasana **145**, **148–9**, *155*,
    220
samadhi (meditative absorption) 5, 8
samtosa (willingness) 4
satya (honesty) 3
sauca (commitment) 3, 4
savasana **18–19**, **22–3**
    backbend practice *223*
    bandha practice *74*
    basis for suptaparivritasana 197
    breath practice *111*
    core practice *56*
    downwards-dog practice *84*
    extension practice *187*
    foundation practice *46*
    full practice *221*
    leg practice *98*
    lunge practice *141*
    quietening practice *225*
    raised leg practice *169*
    relaxation practice *28*
    standing practice *127*
    strengthening practice *211*
    twisting practice *199*
    warrior practice *155*
seated rotation *see* maricyasana
self-enquiry (svadhyaya) 4
sensitivity (ahimsa) 3
shalabasana **203**, **208–9**, *211*, *221*, *222*
shoulderstand, half- *see*
    ardasarvangasana
siddhasana **218–19**
side raised-leg pose *see*
    parsvaikapadasana
side warrior *see* parsvavirabadrasana

sitting cobbler *see* urdvabadakonasana
sitting postures for stillness,
    instructions 216–17
sitting splits *see* urdvakonasana
spine & back 157, 171, 189, 201, 216
spirallic dynamic 65–6, 78–9, 87–8, 113,
    129, 143–4
splits, sitting *see* urdvakonasana
staff pose *see* dandasana
standing fold *see* uttanasana
standing pose *see* tadasana
standing practice *126–7*
stillness 213–17
strengthening practice *210–11*
stretching pose *see* suptahastasana
sukamaricyasana **190**, **192–3**, *198*, *210*,
    221, *222*, *224*
sukasana **20**, **24–5**
    backbend practice *223*
    bandha practice *74*
    basis for other postures 163, 165, 167,
        179
    breath practice *111*
    core practice *56*
    downwards-dog practice *84*
    extension practice *187*
    foundation practice *46*
    full practice *221*
    leg practice *98*
    lunge practice *141*
    quietening practice *225*
    raised leg practice *169*
    relaxation practice *28*
    standing practice *127*
    twisting practice *199*

warrior practice *155*
sun salutation 101
supported lunge *see*
    salambaparsvakonasana
supported side warrior *see*
    salambaparsvavirabadrasana
supported triangle *see*
    salambatrikonasana
supported warrior *see*
    salambavirabadrasana
suptabadakonasana **51**, **54–5**, *56*, *74*
suptahastasana **50**, **52–3**, *56*, *74*
suptaparivritasana **191**, **196–7**, *199*,
    211, *221*, *222*, *225*
svadhyaya (self-enquiry) 4
svanasana **36**, **42–3**, *46*, *56*, *74*, *84*

tadasana **102**, 103, 104, **106–7**, 113
tadottanullola **104**, **109**, *110*
tapas (enthusiasm) 4
throat lock *see* jalandharabandha
triangle pose *see* trikonasana
triangle, revolving *see*
    salambaparivritatrikonasana
triangle, supported *see*
    salambatrikonasana
trikonasana **32–3**, **38–9**, *81*
  bandha practice *74*
  basis for other postures 89, 95, 105,
    113, 139, 143
  breath practice *110*
  core practice *56*

extension practice *186*
foundation practice *46*
full practice *220*
leg practice *98*
lunge practice *140*
raised leg practice *168*
standing practice *126*
strengthening practice *210*
twisting practice *198*
warrior practice *154*
twist, lying *see* suptaparivritasana
twisting pose *see* parivritasana
twisting practice *198–9*
twisting raised-leg pose *see* parivritaika-
    padasana
twists 189

uddiyanabandha 58, 62–3, 66
union, meaning of yoga 1
upwards flying regulator *see* uddiyana-
    bandha
urdvabadakonasana **172**, **178–9**, *187*,
    199, *211*, *221*, *222*
urdvahastullola **103**, **108**
  in practice sequences *110*, *126*, *140*,
    154, *168*, *186*, *198*, *210*, *220*
urdvaikapadasana **159**, **162–3**, *168*,
    186, *198*, *210*, *220*, *224*
urdvakonasana **172**, **176–7**, *186*, *199*,
    211, *221*, *222*
urdvapadottanasa **95**, *98*, 105
utktasana **90**, 96, **97**, 103, 104

in practice sequences *98*, *110*, *126*,
    141, *155*, *168*, *186*, *198*, *210*, *220*
utktullola **103**, **108**
  in practice sequences *110*, *126*, *140*,
    154, *168*, *186*, *198*, *210*, *220*
uttanasana **90**, **96–7**
  in practice sequences *98*, *126*, *141*,
    155, *168*, *186*, *198*, *210*, *220*
  in tadottanullola 104

vinyasa (movement/breath
    synchronization) 8–9, 101

warrior pose *see* hastavirabadrasana
warrior practice *154–5*
warrior, side *see*
    parsvavirabadrasana
warrior, supported *see*
    salambavirabadrasana
warrior, supported side *see*
    salambaparsvavirabadrasana
wheel pose, easy *see* chakrasukasana
willingness (samtosa) 4

yama (attitudes) 3–5, 8, 17, 213, 214
yoga
  bhakti 213
  hatha *see* hatha yoga
  jnana 213
yoga breathing (pranayama) 3, 5, 8, 17,
    213–17
yoga postures *see* asanas

GODFREY DEVEREUX

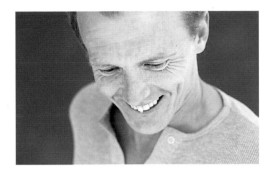

For information about Godfrey's teaching schedule, including teacher training, audio tapes and video tapes, please visit
www.windfireyoga.com

For his interpretation of Patanjali's yoga sutras please visit
yogadarshana.com

Godfrey Devereux teaches Dynamic Yoga on video for the first time.

For more information or to order your copy call 01371 873138 (UK).

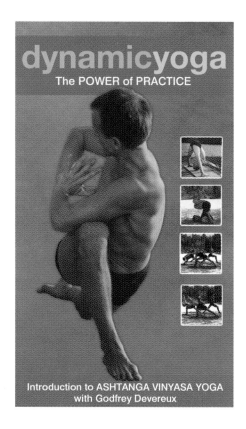

Books by Godfrey Devereux:

Dynamic Yoga

15-minute Yoga

These books are available from all good bookshops or by calling 0870 900 2050 (UK), 1 800 462 6420 (US)
or from Thorsons' website: www.thorsons.com